Minimally Invasive Periodontal Therapy

Clinical Techniques and Visualization Technology

T0176944

Minimally Invasive Periodontal Therapy

Clinical Techniques and Visualization Technology

Edited by

Stephen K. Harrel

Adjunct Professor
Texas A&M University
Baylor College of Dentistry;
Diplomate of the American Board of Periodontology;
President, Texas Medical and Dental Designs, LLC;
Private Practice
Dallas, Texas, USA

Thomas G. Wilson Jr.

Diplomate of the American Board of Periodontology;
Clinical Associate Professor
University of Texas at San Antonio;
Private Practice
Dallas, Texas, USA

WILEY Blackwell

This edition first published 2015 © 2015 by John Wiley & Sons, Inc.

Editorial offices

1606 Golden Aspen Drive, Suites 103 and 104, Ames, Iowa 50010, USA

The Atrium, Southern Gate, Chichester, West Sussex, PO19 8SQ, UK

9600 Garsington Road, Oxford, OX4 2DQ, UK

For details of our global editorial offices, for customer services and for information about how to apply for permission to reuse the copyright material in this book please see our website at www.wiley.com/wiley-blackwell.

Library of Congress Cataloging-in-Publication Data

Harrel, Stephen K., author.

 Minimally invasive periodontal therapy : clinical techniques and visualization technology / Stephen K. Harrel, Thomas G. Wilson, Jr.

  p. ; cm.

 Includes bibliographical references and index.

 ISBN 978-1-118-60762-6 (pbk.)

 I. Wilson, Thomas G., Jr., author. II. Title.

 [DNLM: 1. Periodontal Diseases–surgery. 2. Surgical Procedures, Minimally Invasive–instrumentation. 3. Surgical Procedures, Minimally Invasive–methods. WU 240]

 RK361

 617.6′32–dc23

2014033178

A catalogue record for this book is available from the British Library.

Wiley also publishes its books in a variety of electronic formats. Some content that appears in print may not be available in electronic books.

Cover image: Front cover inset: Reproduced with permission of Perioscopy Incorporated;
          Back cover inset: Courtesy of Dr. Francisco Rivera-Hidalgo.

Set in 10.5/12.5pt Palatino by SPi Publisher Services, Pondicherry, India

Printed in Singapore by C.O.S. Printers Pte Ltd

1 2015

Contents

Contributors   vii
Introduction   ix
About the Companion Website   xi

1 Overview of Minimally Invasive Therapy   1
   Stephen K. Harrel and Thomas G. Wilson Jr.

2 Visualization for Minimally Invasive Periodontal Therapy:
   An Overview   3
   Stephen K. Harrel

3 Ultrasonic Endoscopic Periodontal Debridement   13
   John Y. Kwan and Suzanne M. Newkirk

4 Endoscope Use in Daily Hygiene Practice   55
   Kara Webb and Angela R. Anderson

5 The Use of the Dental Endoscope and Videoscope for Diagnosis
   and Treatment of Peri-Implant Diseases   65
   Thomas G. Wilson Jr.

6 Development of Minimally Invasive Periodontal
   Surgical Techniques   77
   Stephen K. Harrel

7 The MIS and V-MIS Surgical Procedure   81
   Stephen K. Harrel

8   Minimally Invasive Surgical Technique and Modified-MIST
    in Periodontal Regeneration   117
    Pierpaolo Sandro Cortellini

9   Minimally Invasive Soft Tissue Grafting   143
    Edward P. Allen and Lewis C. Cummings

10 Future Potential for Minimally Invasive Periodontal Therapy   165
    Stephen K. Harrel and Thomas G. Wilson Jr.

Index   171

Contributors

Edward P. Allen
Adjunct Professor
Department of Periodontics, Texas
A&M University Baylor College of
Dentistry

Director
Center for Advanced Dental
Education

Private Practice
Dallas, TX, USA

Angela R. Anderson, RDH
Private Practice
Dallas, TX, USA

Pierpaolo Sandro Cortellini, MD, DDS
Treasurer of Academia Toscana di
Ricerca Odontostomatologica (ATRO)
Firenze

Private Practice
Firenze, Italy

Board member of European Research
Group on Periodontology
(ERGOPERIO)
Berne, Switzerland

Lewis C. Cummings
Associate Clinical Professor
University of Texas Dental School
Houston, TX, USA

University of Nebraska College of
Dentistry
Lincoln, NE, USA

Center for Advanced Dental
Education
Dallas, TX, USA

American Institute of Implant
Dentistry
Washington, DC, USA

Stephen K. Harrel
Adjunct Professor
Texas A&M University
Baylor College of Dentistry

Diplomate of the American Board of
Periodontology

President
Texas Medical and Dental Designs, LLC

Private Practice
Dallas, TX, USA

John Y. Kwan, DDS
Associate Clinical Professor
University of California –
San Francisco
School of Dentistry
San Francisco, CA, USA

Suzanne M. Newkirk, RDH
Private Practice
Lakemont, GA, USA

Kara Webb, RDH
Private Practice
Dallas, TX, USA

Thomas G. Wilson Jr.
Diplomate of the American Board of
Periodontology

Private Practice
Dallas, TX, USA

Introduction

Minimally invasive treatment is a major advancement in dental therapy and is rapidly becoming part of the average dentist's daily practice. These innovations range from cavity preparation through surgical modalities. The extent of this radical advancement can be illustrated by changes in periodontal therapy. It was traditionally necessary to elevate large mucogingival flaps for access to underlying structures. These procedures often resulted in esthetic deformities, food impaction, and increased thermal sensitivity. The innovations described in this text detail approaches that stand in marked contrast to traditional methods. Minimally invasive methods for periodontal treatment routinely yield long-term reductions of probing depths and increased clinical attachment levels that exceed those reported for traditional approaches. In addition, minimal thermal hypersensitivity and no gingival recession have been reported. One of the greatest advantages to the clinician is the increased patient acceptance and satisfaction with minimal encroachment versus traditional approaches.

This text will allow the reader to understand minimally invasive periodontal procedures and how they can benefit the reader's practice. It is directed toward any therapist who treats periodontal diseases. Specifics concerning the application and use of various forms of these approaches will be detailed. This text explores areas far advanced from traditional methods. It will give the reader significant information on the advantages of the application of minimally invasive procedures to their daily practice.

About the Companion Website

This book is accompanied by a companion website:

www.wiley.com/go/harrel/minimallyinvasive

The website includes videos showing:

Placement of the endoscope into the sulcus
Subgingival Caries
Root Fracture
Calculus
Open Margin
Endodontic Perforation
Resorption
Excess Cement on an Implant

1 Overview of Minimally Invasive Therapy

Stephen K. Harrel and Thomas G. Wilson Jr.

The definition of a minimally invasive procedure has been debated in medicine since the term was first coined in an editorial in the *British Journal of Surgery* in 1990 [1]. Initial descriptions of small incision surgeries were usually based on the method or instrument that was used to visualize the surgical site. Examples of this would be a microsurgical procedure where the surgical site was visualized using a surgical microscope or a laparoscopic procedure where the abdominal procedure was visualized using a laparoscopic endoscope. Because the technology being used for small incision surgery continued to evolve rapidly and often the instrumentation for visualization of a particular procedure changed over time, the term "minimally invasive surgery" was suggested. This is a more global term that need not be changed as the technology evolves. Over time, a definition was accepted which states that minimally invasive surgery is a surgical technique that uses smaller incisions to perform a surgical procedure that previously required larger incisions and achieves equal or superior results compared with the traditional surgical approach [2]. This definition separates the description of the surgical procedure from the technology used for visualizing the surgery. This broad-based definition is currently accepted in most medical fields.

A significant portion of this text will explore periodontal therapeutic approaches that are markedly different from traditional techniques. Some of these techniques clearly fit the medical definition of minimally invasive surgery. These include the

Minimally Invasive Periodontal Therapy: Clinical Techniques and Visualization Technology, First Edition.
Edited by Stephen K. Harrel and Thomas G. Wilson Jr.
© 2015 John Wiley & Sons, Inc. Published 2015 by John Wiley & Sons, Inc.
Companion Website: www.wiley.com/go/harrel/minimallyinvasive

surgical approaches where very small incisions using a videoscope are used to treat periodontal bone loss or to treat soft tissue deficiencies. Some of the techniques described do not fit the usually accepted definition of minimally invasive surgery. An example is closed gingival scaling and root planing using a dental endoscope. However, the editors feel that this procedure clearly belongs in the broader area of minimally invasive therapy.

The scientific documentation on minimally invasive techniques is approaching a critical mass. The number of papers that document very favorable results from minimally invasive surgical and nonsurgical periodontal procedures is increasing and have been generated from multiple sources. This is a critical factor for minimally invasive therapies to become a mainstream and, eventually, the dominant therapeutic approach. At the same time, the devices for performing MIS are becoming more widely available. This combination of positive scientific evidence and advances in technology will allow rapid advancement in the field.

This book briefly describes some of the early applications of this philosophy, how the technologies for performing minimally invasive procedures have evolved, and how the current techniques have reached their present form. The book also covers in detail the state of the art in minimally invasive periodontal therapy. This includes a description of the techniques, a discussion of the currently used technology, as well as clinical case studies. Chapter 10 explores possible futures for the treatment of periodontal disease that may take us far beyond our current concepts of what is "minimal" in our treatment approaches.

References

1. Wickham, J. & Fitzpatric, J.M. (1990) Minimally invasive surgery [Editorial]. *British Journal of Surgery*, **77**, 721–722.
2. Hunter, J.G. & Sackier, J.M. (1993) Minimally invasive high tech surgery: Into the 21st century. In: J.G. Hunter & J.M. Sackier (eds), *Minimally Invasive Surgery*, pp. 3–6. McGraw-Hill, New York.

2 Visualization for Minimally Invasive Periodontal Therapy: An Overview

Stephen K. Harrel

The increasing popularity of minimally invasive procedures has been driven in part by advancements in technology that have allowed procedures to be performed through smaller access openings and by the reduced morbidity and improved efficacy seen as a result of these technologies. The most critical advancements in technology are in the area of visualization. The key to performing minimally invasive procedures is the ability to adequately see the site and, therefore, the ability to successfully complete the indicated surgical manipulations. With enhanced visualization, outcomes are improved.

Traditional closed subgingival scaling and root planing is the most frequently used approach for treating inflammatory periodontal diseases. This approach allows no direct visualization of the treatment site. Treatment end points are based on the tactile sense of the operator using various instruments. The operator is forced to determine by palpation alone if the root surface has been debrided of calculus and if root roughness has been removed. Because of a lack of a tactical "feel," it is impossible for the operator to determine by palpation if any existing biofilm has been completely removed. The process of determining a clinically ideal end point is complicated by factors such as burnished calculus and various root anomalies that give a less-than-smooth feel to the root. While closed root planing has been shown to routinely improve periodontal health, it has also been shown that the end result is often a root surface with some residual calculus. It was found that root surfaces treated with these traditional methods when subsequently

Minimally Invasive Periodontal Therapy: Clinical Techniques and Visualization Technology, First Edition.
Edited by Stephen K. Harrel and Thomas G. Wilson Jr.
© 2015 John Wiley & Sons, Inc. Published 2015 by John Wiley & Sons, Inc.
Companion Website: www.wiley.com/go/harrel/minimallyinvasive

viewed either with the endoscope or the videoscope routinely reveal areas of retained calculus and biofilm. Thus, the lack of visualization in traditional closed approaches frequently results in subsequent periodontal breakdown and frequently leads to further treatment often including surgery.

Traditional periodontal surgery was developed to allow for access and visualization of the surgical site. One of the most commonly performed traditional periodontal surgical procedures is open-flap debridement. This approach allows for visualization of the root surface and periodontal defect. The incisions traditionally used to provide visualization often extend over many teeth and often include areas that have little or no periodontal damage. Elevation of these large flaps frequently leads to post-surgical root exposure, areas of food impaction, and thermal sensitivity as well as esthetic deformities.

Minimally invasive periodontal therapy is designed to access and visualize only the areas that require periodontal treatment using the smallest incision possible. This has been made possible by technologic advances for visualization without the necessity of large incisions and flap elevation. This chapter explores the options currently available for visualization. The advantages and disadvantages of each will be discussed.

Visualization for closed root planing procedures

The very nature of closed root planing demands that visualization of the treatment site uses a visualization technology that can be placed into an intact pocket without a surgical incision. To date, there is a single device, the periodontal endoscope which was developed in the 1990s, that will allow for this approach [1] (Figure 2.1). This endoscope consists of glass fibers contained within a plastic

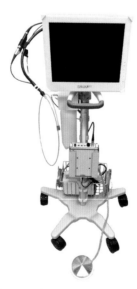

Figure 2.1 The glass fiber endoscope for use in nonsurgical minimally invasive periodontal therapy is shown. Source: Courtesy of Dr. John Kwan.

disposable sheath with a small stainless steel tube, and a sealed sapphire lens. The stainless steel tube is retained in a handheld dental instrument that allows the fibers and lens to be directed into the periodontal pocket without flap elevation. Some of the glass fibers direct light into the subgingival environment. Other glass fibers capture an image of this space. The image is returned to an external camera that displays it on a monitor. The operator can directly view the treatment area by looking at the monitor that allows them to determine the need for and efficacy of efforts to remove root-bound deposits.

The currently available glass fiber endoscope is less than 1 mm in diameter. It contains several thousand individual optical glass fibers. It is considered flexible because some amount of bending and flexing is possible. However, care must be taken to avoid significant bending of the fibers to reduce the probability of fracture. Typically, even with care, some of the individual glass fibers will break with use. As fractures occur, there will be some degradation of the amount of light that reaches the surgical site, and the image returned to the external camera will be degraded. The image will continue to degrade with use until the endoscope fibers have to be replaced. This degradation and the need for replacement can be a significant factor in the expense of using a periodontal endoscope.

A sheath to cover the glass fibers is necessary because the fibers cannot be sterilized. The sheath comes sterilized and the endoscope is fully contained within the sterile sheath (Figure 2.2). The sheath also acts as a conduit for liquid that flows into the sulcus to keep the treatment site clear of blood and debris. Without a constant flow of liquid, the optics of the endoscope would rapidly become fouled and impossible to use. The surgical sheath is a one-time use item that adds a moderate amount of expense to its use.

The currently available glass fiber endoscope is the only device that allows visualization of the root surface without the necessity of surgical access. As such, this instrument is unique, and there is no other available alternative for visualization during closed root planing. There are concerns about the endoscope that have limited its acceptance for routine periodontal treatments. Among these is the lack of clarity of the image delivered to the monitor. Most of the lack of clarity is because of the limited number of glass fibers available to transmit the picture. More fibers

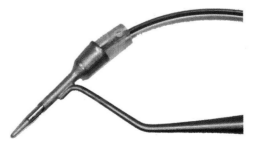

Figure 2.2   The single-use sterile disposable sheath for the glass fiber endoscope is shown. Source: Courtesy of Dr. John Kwan.

would increase the diameter of the device and limit its use without flap elevation. Another contributor to the lack of clarity is the amount of debris suspended in the irrigating liquid. The image can be enhanced by moving the instrument over the root surface and causing the debris in the sulcus to be flushed by the flow of irrigant. In addition, the learning curve for this instrument can be quite steep.

Potential improvements for nonsurgical visualization are numerous. The first goal would be to improve the picture quality. This might be accomplished by an increase in the number of optical fibers. This would allow a greater number of fibers to bring light to the sulcus as well as provide more fibers to transmit the picture to the monitor. Another possible improvement would be to have a better method to keep the treatment area clear of blood and debris. The liquid that constantly flows through the sulcus tends to rapidly become cloudy. This further limits visualization of the treatment area. Any improvement in visualization should include making the endoscope more reliable and less fragile.

Current technology makes it difficult to further improve the glass fiber endoscope. An increase in the number of fibers for optical transmission carries with it the necessity of making the endoscope larger, which in turn would make the placement of the endoscope in the sulcus more difficult, painful, and traumatic. At some point, it may be possible to use smaller fibers that would overcome some of these technical difficulties. It is more likely that improvements in videoscope technology will overcome the present problems. This is true because a videoscope utilizes a tiny camera that is placed directly in the treatment area and does not depend on glass fibers to transmit an image. Unfortunately, the smallest currently available camera is still too large for application to nonsurgical root planing. A videoscope is currently being used for minimally invasive periodontal surgery and will be described later in this chapter.

Visualization for minimally invasive periodontal surgery

Small incision periodontal surgery has traditionally used either a surgical microscope or surgical telescopes (often referred to as loupes). Both of these instruments offer magnification, and usually have some type of light source integrated into the device. However, both of these devices have significant limitations in their application to periodontal minimally invasive surgery.

Surgical telescopes (loupes)

In the early reports of minimally invasive surgery, surgical telescopes were used for magnification [2]. Surgical telescopes are magnifiers that usually clip on or are affixed to eyeglasses (Figure 2.3). Surgical telescopes work by magnifying a portion of the surgical field. Looking over the top of the telescope allows the surgeon to view a larger surgical field with no magnification. Magnification with surgical telescopes is usually from 2× to 7.5×. The most commonly used telescopes are in

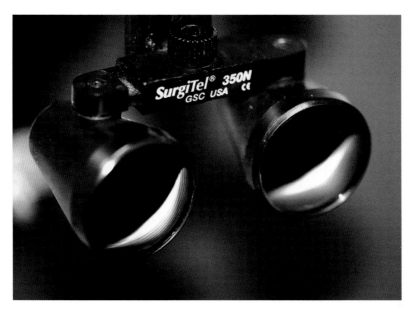

Figure 2.3   A surgical telescope or loupe with an integral light is shown. Source: Courtesy of Dr. Jonathan Blansett.

the range of 3× to 5×. Surgical telescopes also come in a range of focal distances that allow the surgeon to sit in a comfortable upright position while maintaining focus on the surgical site. The focal length of the telescopes is selected to fit the surgeon's personal preferences. Often, a high intensity light will be integrated into surgical telescopes. The light can be halogen or LED and can usually be focused to a very narrow diameter. The ability to place a bright focused light on the field that is magnified is a major advantage when small incisions surgeries are performed.

One of the advantages of surgical telescopes over surgical microscopes (see below) is that the surgeon is in complete control of where the magnification and illumination is centered. This means that the surgeon can look quickly at several areas within the surgical field without having to move any external piece of equipment such as a surgical microscope. In addition, if the patient moves, redirecting of the magnification is the natural movement of the surgeon's head. The use of surgical telescopes has become standard in many areas of dentistry. Often, a surgeon who is performing minimally invasive periodontal procedures is already familiar and comfortable with the use of telescopes that makes the use of this form of magnification a logical first step in transitioning from traditional periodontal surgery to minimally invasive procedures.

Surgical telescopes have several disadvantages over other methods available for magnification. The most obvious is that much greater magnification is available with other devices. These alternate devices generally have magnification potential in the 10× to 60× range. Surgical telescopes that magnify beyond the 7.5× range can be heavy and difficult to use. Another disadvantage of surgical telescopes is the fact that the surgeon is limited to direct vision. This means that there will be blind spots where a mirror is necessary to see the surgical area of interest. An example is the distal of a second molar or an interproximal site. This is a disadvantage that surgical telescope shares with the surgical microscope. The endoscope and videoscope offer significant advantages in these areas.

In summary, surgical telescopes are an excellent, but limited tool, for minimally invasive surgery. They are particularly useful for a surgeon just starting to make the transition from traditional periodontal surgery to a minimally invasive approach.

Surgical microscope

The surgical microscope has been in use for over 50 years (Figure 2.4). It was developed and first used for surgery of the inner ear. Since that time, the surgical microscope has been applied to many types of surgeries. This device offers the advantages of high magnification, a bright light source, and an open field for surgery. The open field is based on the relatively long focal distance between the microscope objective stage and the surgical site. This allows the placement of instruments into the magnified field of the microscope.

The surgical microscope is a relatively large instrument that either requires a bulky and heavy stand if the microscope is designed to be moved between treatment rooms, or requires a reinforced ceiling or wall mount if it is to be permanently installed in an operatory. The need for a large and stable mounting adds considerably to the cost of this relatively expensive instrument.

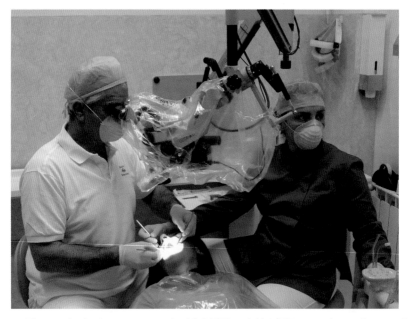

Figure 2.4 The surgical microscope used with MIST and M-MIST procedures. Source: Courtesy of Dr. Pierpaolo Cortellini.

In periodontal surgery, the surgical microscope has found frequent application for the placement of soft tissue grafts and in periodontal plastic surgeries [3]. The anterior segment of the mouth and the facial aspect of the anterior teeth and gingiva are the areas where the surgical microscope is most easily used. This segment of the mouth allows for an unimpeded straight-line view of the surgical field. The surgical microscope has allowed for many improvements in the handling of facial tissues and the suturing of tissues during esthetic procedures.

The surgical microscope has also been used during the development of the minimally invasive surgical technique procedures (MIST and M-MIST) [4,5]. In most reported cases, the MIST procedures have used a facial flap access, which may have been influenced by using the surgical microscope. Using surgical microscope in the posterior and in lingual areas requires a great deal of skill and the use of mirrors to compensate for the straight-line viewing field of the surgical microscope.

Another concern with the surgical microscope is the necessity to refocus the microscope if the patient moves. In general, it is not possible to move the microscope to compensate for small movements of the patient such as swallowing or normal microhead movements. It is usually simpler to return the patient to their previous position. This can often be carried out with minimal disruption of the procedure; but if the patient is uncooperative, nervous, sedated, or has difficulty holding a fixed position, this can add considerably to the length of time necessary to perform a procedure.

In summary, the surgical microscope provides good magnification and light, but it requires a great deal of operator skill and patient cooperation for successful use. Many operators have had difficulty in adapting to the use of the surgical microscope for periodontal procedures. However, those who have persevered in the use of the surgical microscope have been able to use it for many very technically demanding procedures and for surgical procedures using very small minimal-access incisions.

Surgical videoscope

A traditional medical endoscope consists of a stainless steel tube containing lenses that carry the image from the tip of the endoscope to a camera that is outside of the surgical field. The external camera then transfers the image to a monitor. The flexible glass endoscope designed for nonsurgical periodontal treatment that was described earlier also transfers an image to an external camera that places the image on a monitor. The videoscope has a different method of transferring the image to the monitor. With a videoscope a very small camera is placed at the end of the scope and the camera is placed within the surgical field. The image is then transferred to the monitor by an electrical signal through a wire. This eliminates any degradations of the image that might occur during transmission of the image from the surgical site through optical fibers to an external camera. In general, the image viewed on the videoscope monitor is in true color and is of much higher quality than that obtained with a glass fiber endoscope.

A videoscope designed for the nonsurgical exploration of the kidney has recently been modified for use in videoscope-assisted minimally invasive periodontal surgery (V-MIS) (Figure 2.5). The modifications consist of the adaptation of the camera end of the insertion tube of the videoscope to a handle that allows the surgeon to place the camera into the minimally invasive periodontal surgical access opening. Incorporated into the handle is a small carbon fiber retractor that is designed to retract the very small flaps associated with V-MIS (Figure 2.6). This carbon fiber retractor can be rotated in a manner that will allow the surgeon to retract V-MIS flaps on the buccal or lingual aspect of the periodontal defect.

As with all endoscopic or videoscopic instruments, a major concern is keeping blood and surgical debris from obscuring the optics of the instrument. Without an effective method to keep the optics clear, it is impossible to use an endoscope or videoscope. It is not practical to continuously flow water over the lens of the videoscope, nor is it possible to keep an open surgical field filled with liquid as is used for nonsurgical minimally invasive treatment of periodontal disease with the glass fiber endoscope. A technology that uses a constant flow of surgical gases or air over the lens has been developed to overcome this problem during periodontal use of the videoscope (Figure 2.7). This technology is described as

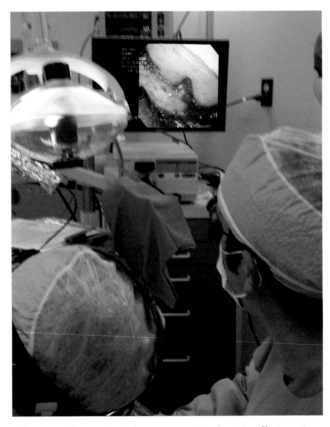

Figure 2.5 The videoscope for use in videoscope-assisted minimally invasive surgery (V-MIS) is shown in use. Source: Courtesy of Dr. Francisco Rivera-Hidalgo.

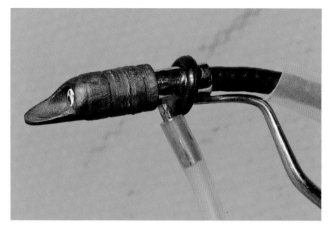

Figure 2.6   The handpiece for holding the videoscope used in V-MIS. The rotating carbon fiber retractor is shown surrounding the camera of the videoscope.

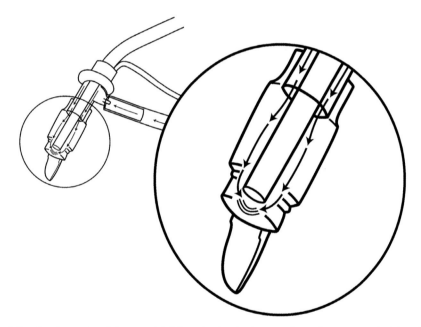

Figure 2.7   A schematic of the gas shielding device is shown. The videoscope is held within a "shield" of turbulent surgical gases to avoid fouling or fogging of the videoscope optics.

gas shielding of the optics. Its application to a videoscope used for periodontal MIS procedures allows the videoscope to be used continuously without the need to clean or clear the optics. The modified videoscope with gas shielding has been used in a university-based study of minimally invasive periodontal surgery. Preliminary results have shown good visualization with improved attachment levels and pocket depths that are similar or improved over other published results for small incision surgeries [6,7]. The use of the videoscope appears to allow for a reduction in post-surgical recession.

Summary

The improvements in the techniques for performing all minimally invasive surgeries have been driven by improvements in the technology for visualization of the surgical site. As visualization has improved over time, it has been possible to make smaller incisions for surgical procedures and to perform more complete root debridement in nonsurgical periodontal procedures. It is probable that there will be a continuation of improvements in visualization technology, which will drive changes and improvements in future surgical techniques.

References

1. Stambaugh, R.V., Myers, G., Ebling, W., Beckman, & B. Stambaugh, K. (2002) Endoscope visualization of the subgingival dental sulcus and tooth root surface. *Journal of Periodontology*, **73**, 374–382.
2. Harrel, S.K. (1999) A minimally invasive surgical approach for periodontal regeneration: Surgical technique and observations. *Journal of Periodontology*, **70**, 1547–1557.
3. Tibbetts, L.S. & Shanelelc, D. (1998) Periodontal microsurgery. *Dental Clinics of North America*, **42** (**2**),339–359.
4. Cortellini, P. & Tonetti, M.S. (2007) A minimally invasive surgical technique with an enamel matrix derivative in the regenerative treatment of intra-bony defects: A novel approach to limit morbidity. *Journal of Clinical Periodontology*, **34**, 87–93.
5. Cortellini, P. & Tonetti, M.S. (2009) Improved wound stability with a modified minimally invasive surgical technique in the regenerative treatment of isolated interdental intrabony defects. *Journal of Clinical Periodontology*, **36**, 157–163.
6. Harrel, S.K., Rivera-Hidalgo, F. & Abraham, C. (2012) Tissue resistance to soft tissue emphysema during minimally invasive surgery. *Journal of Contemporary Dental Practice*, **13** (**6**), 886–891.
7. Harrel, S.K., Wilson, T.G. Jr. & Rivera-Hidalgo, F. (2013) A videoscope for use in minimally invasive periodontal surgery. *Journal of Clinical Periodontology* **40**, 868–874.

3 Ultrasonic Endoscopic Periodontal Debridement

John Y. Kwan and Suzanne M. Newkirk

The purpose of this chapter is to identify the benefits of minimally invasive periodontal therapy utilizing endoscopic technology that provides real-time video magnification, enabling clinicians to diagnose and treat periodontal disease subgingivally and nonsurgically under direct visualization (Figure 3.1).

Introduction

The use of the endoscope has become accepted in most medical surgical disciplines. Today, minimally invasive procedures routinely result in rapid wound healing, fewer complications, and shorter recovery times [1]. The periodontal endoscope consists of a 1mm diameter, 1m long, flexible endoscope/camera attached to a dental instrument referred to as an endoscopic "explorer," which carries a lens attached to a fiber-optic cable that can be placed subgingivally and provides the clinician with visualization of the subgingival environment.

The images are immediately displayed on a chairside monitor (real-time video) and magnified 24–48 times, disclosing minute details, such as caries, root fractures, perforations, resorption, biofilm, and calculus, that previously may have been undetectable. The authors call this illumination and magnification of the subgingival environment a "microvisual" approach.

Minimally Invasive Periodontal Therapy: Clinical Techniques and Visualization Technology, First Edition.
Edited by Stephen K. Harrel and Thomas G. Wilson Jr.
© 2015 John Wiley & Sons, Inc. Published 2015 by John Wiley & Sons, Inc.
Companion Website: www.wiley.com/go/harrel/minimallyinvasive

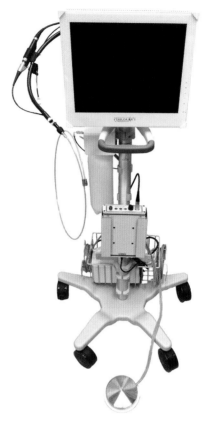

Figure 3.1 The Perioscopy System. Source: Reproduced with permission of Perioscopy Incorporated.

Dental endoscopy has been shown to reveal deposits so small that they cannot be seen during traditional periodontal surgery, even with a surgical microscope or dental magnifying loupes [2]. Dental microscopes have magnifications from 2 × to 20 ×. At the highest magnifications, the slightest movement can affect the image. This is because of the long distance between the objective lens of the microscope and the actual image in the mouth. In addition, visualization on the internal aspects of the dentition as well as on the distal of posterior teeth is limited. The periodontal endoscope is intimately close to the root surface; therefore, the image easily stays within the focal depth of field. With fiber-optic illumination and high magnification the dental endoscope allows for visualization of root surfaces, the inner aspects of most furcations, and into bony defects that cannot be seen with any other device except surgically with the dental video scope [2]. Endoscopic periodontal debridement is the only nonsurgical minimally invasive, real-time video technology available for the treatment of periodontal disease.

Indications for the use of the endoscopic technique

Candidates for endoscopy include patients being treated for the following:

- initial periodontal therapy;
- sites that have not responded to traditional nonsurgical debridement;
- maintenance patients with chronically inflamed, or increasing probing depths;
- residual probing depths in maintenance patients who refuse surgical therapy and/or where surgery is contraindicated for medical, or esthetic reasons;
- suspected subgingival pathology such as caries, root fractures, perforations, or resorption.

There are several endoscopic systems available for dental use. The ones described here—the DV2 Perioscopy System and the Perioscopy System— are used for providing nonsurgical periodontal therapy and minimally invasive diagnosis. These systems have six main features:

Components

1	2	3	4	5	6
Camera light source	Monitor	Endoscope fiber	Sheath	Explorer	Water delivery device

1. The DV2 Perioscopy System master control unit (MCU) camera and light source provide real-time video images. The light source is an arc lamp that creates intense, focused light fiber optically delivered to the working field.

   The Perioscopy System utilizes a CCD/LED camera and light coupling to provide imaging and illumination from the endoscope fiber to the monitor through a controller. The controller has window, gain control, white balance, and illumination settings that are optimized for dental endoscopy. A "handpiece" contains the camera and LED along with a focus knob (Figure 3.2).

2. The DV2 Perioscopy System color LCD video monitor provides real-time, detailed color images of the procedure site as viewed by the attached endoscope (Figure 3.3).

   The Perioscopy System medical grade monitor provides high definition, real-time video imaging received from the dental endoscope. The image is 25% larger, and the resolution is a significant improvement over the DV2 System (Figure 3.4).

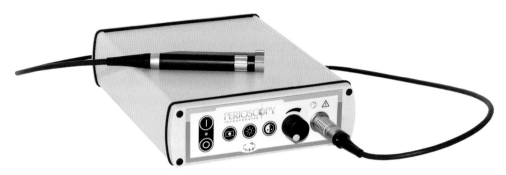

Figure 3.2 Perioscopy System Camera/LED/controller. Source: Reproduced with permission of Perioscopy Incorporated.

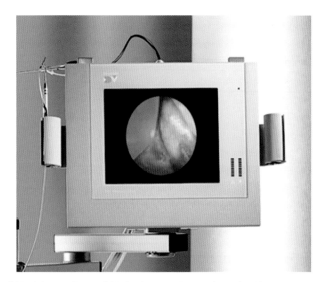

Figure 3.3 The DV2 Master Control Unit. Source: Reproduced with permission of Perioscopy Incorporated.

3. The dental endoscope (or fiber) is a device for use with the dental endoscope family of dental instruments. The fiber consists of a very slender, flexible shaft containing both imaging and illumination capabilities. When inserted into the dental endoscopic sheath and then the endoscopic explorers, the endoscope fiber provides detailed and highly magnified images of the diagnostic and/or treatment site (Figure 3.5).

The microscope lens system enlarges the image obtained by the fiber-optic probe and creates intense, focused light that is fiber optically delivered to

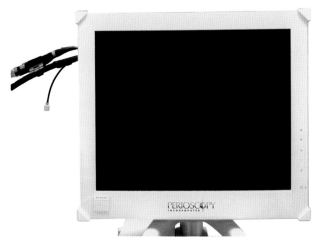

Figure 3.4   The perioscopy system medical grade monitor. Source: Reproduced with permission of Perioscopy Incorporated.

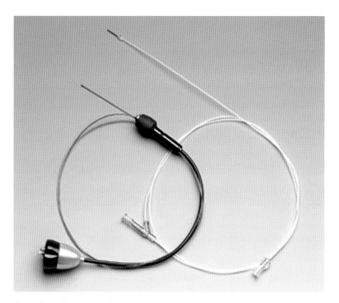

Figure 3.5   The dental endoscope (fiber) and sheath. Source: Reproduced with permission of Perioscopy Incorporated.

the working field. This reusable fiber-optic endoscope is 1 mm in diameter and 1 m long with containing 20 different fibers. The quartz sleeve encased fiber-optic probe is made of 19, 125 μm light guides that deliver light to the working field. They surround a 10,000-pixel image guide made up of fused 2 μm fibers to capture the image. The end of the probe has a hand microp-olished gradient index lens and provides a 3-mm-wide field of view. The working depth of field allows for focus from 2 to 6 mm from the tip, with 4.5 mm being optimum. The magnification is 24×–48× depending on the closeness to the lens.

The fiber does not require routine sterilization when used with the endoscopic sheath.

4. The sheath: A single-use disposable endoscopic sheath is designed to deliver water irrigation to keep the endoscope lens clear, eliminate the need to sterilize or disinfect the fiber between cases, and to provide a significantly longer fiber life. Bilumen construction consist of clear tubing that completely covers the endoscopic fiber and blue tubing that carries water irrigation to the working site (Figure 3.6).

Each sterile sheath has a sapphire window, a window cell (a stainless steel tube with sapphire lens), a precision tip seal, and dual Luer–Lock connectors for water and fiber connections. These elements create a fluid-tight seal that ensures accurate positioning to the working tip of the endoscopic explorer (Figure 3.7).

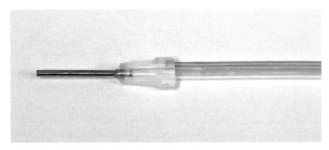

Figure 3.6 Single use, sterile endoscopic sheath. Source: Reproduced with permission of Perioscopy Incorporated.

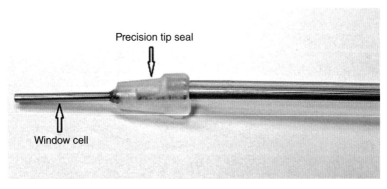

Figure 3.7 Endoscopic sheath highlighting the precision tip seal and window cell. Source: Reproduced with permission of Perioscopy Incorporated.

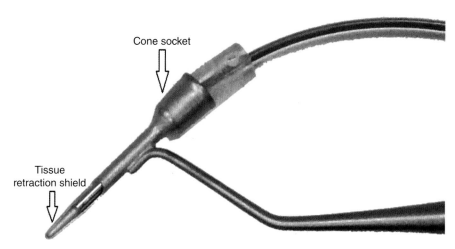

Cone socket

Tissue
retraction shield

Figure 3.8 Endoscopic explorer tissue retraction shield. Source: Reproduced with permission of Perioscopy Incorporated.

5. The fiber is placed into a sterile sheath and is then placed into an endoscopic explorer. The fiber–sheath–explorer complex is then placed into the sulcus by the clinician for subgingival viewing.

Dental endoscopic explorers are sterilizable dental instruments that hold the sheath/fiber complex, allowing for intraoral use.
     The endoscopic explorer has a shield that deflects the pocket soft tissue away from the camera lens, creating visual access space to the root surface (Figure 3.8).

6. A pressurized, self-contained water delivery device is attached to the cart of the dental endoscopic system, and it not only provides a constant source of lavage into the pocket during an endoscopic procedure but also keeps the lens free from debris such as blood and tissue, providing a clear video image. The water delivery device connects to a standard in-office air line and operates by a rheostat pedal through an air-operated valve (Figure 3.9).

Exploring the subgingival environment

When the dental endoscope is used subgingivally in a periodontal pocket, a loose film adhering to the tooth is frequently observed. This material is easily disturbed by the shield on the endoscopic explorer. During scaling of the subgingival root surface, this film loses adherence and is washed away by irrigation water flowing from the endoscope probe [3]. It is assumed to be biofilm (Figure 3.10).
     Typically, the gingival wall of the healthy sulcus is light pink in color, indicating health. In disease, islands of dark red color blotch the pocket wall. These areas vary from a slight color change to deep red with an erythematous

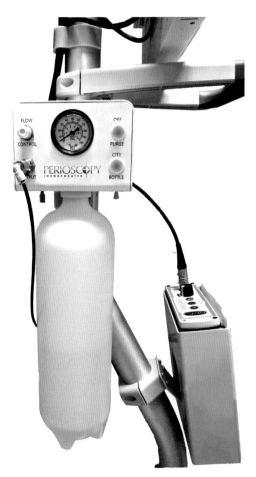

Figure 3.9 Endoscopic water delivery device. Source: Reproduced with permission of Perioscopy Incorporated.

appearance and may be discrete or diffuse. In addition, these red areas have been shown to be primarily associated with calculus covered with biofilm, not biofilm alone, which emphasizes the role of calculus in the pathophysiology of this chronic inflammatory periodontal disease [3]. This also argues strongly for removal of all calculus deposits seen subgingivally to reduce or eliminate inflammation.

Because of bright fiber-optic illumination, calculus found on the dental root structure commonly shows up as gold, yellow, or white. Calculus deposits may range from small isolated flecks, or islands, to thick, continuous layers [3]. Prior to periodontal endoscopy, visualization and more thorough debridement of the subgingival environment were only accomplished through surgical intervention via open-flap debridement. Even after traditional surgery, deposits of subgingival calculus have been shown to remain [4]. The ability to clearly visualize and remove calculus with nonsurgical therapy is a major advantage of periodontal endoscopy.

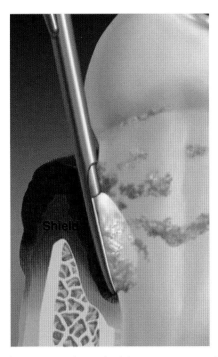

Figure 3.10 The dental endoscopic explorer shield retracting tissue from the pocket wall to expose the root surface for viewing. Source: Reproduced with permission of Perioscopy Incorporated.

Factors affecting instrumentation in non-surgical debridement include:

Deposit/ calculus	Instrument access	Root morphology considerations	Anatomical considerations/ other
Amount	Narrow deep pockets	Bi and tri-furcated teeth	Small mouth
Tenacity	Curved roots	Concavities	Muscular tongues
Location	Close root proximity	Line angles	Tight cheeks and lips
	Over contoured restorations	Depressions	Gaggers
	Distal aspects of second or third molars	Developmental grooves	Patient cooperation
			Operator experience

The primary goal of periodontal therapy is the reduction or elimination of inflammation. Traditionally, this is accomplished through removal of subgingival tooth-borne accretions using non-surgical and/or surgical treatment modalities [5]. Because periodontal pathogens reside in deep subgingival sites and also colonize supragingival plaque on the tongue dorsum and other oral sites, the control of destructive periodontal diseases may warrant a comprehensive antimicrobial approach that targets periodontal pathogens in various ecological niches of the oral cavity [5]. Scaling and root planing (with or without periodontal surgery) along with proper personal oral hygiene constitute the primary approach to controlling periodontopathogens [5].

However, traditional nonsurgical periodontal therapy provided in a closed environment utilizing a combination of hand instrumentation and powered instruments has been shown to be both time consuming and technically difficult to perform [4]. Even very experienced clinicians may be deceived by tactilely smooth surfaces achieved by instrumentation and assume the root surfaces are free of deposits. Endoscopic evaluation of root surfaces that have undergone scaling in a closed manner with various powered instruments, especially under low power, consistently reveals retained burnished calculus on the root surface ranging in size from large, smooth, and flat sheets, to small, flat "islands." These residual deposits are usually located in furcations, developmental depressions, at line angles and around the cementoenamel junction [2].

In an evaluation of the effectiveness of traditional subgingival scaling and root planing related to depth of pocket and type of teeth, results demonstrated a high correlation between the percentage of residual calculus and probing depth. It was shown that probing depths less than 3 mm were the easiest sites for effective scaling and root planing, probing depths between 3 and 5 mm were more difficult to completely remove calculus and biofilm, and probing depths deeper than 5 mm were the most difficult sites. Tooth type did not influence the results [6]. Endoscopic examination revealed residual burnished calculus in 100% of pockets and furcations that bleed upon probing and that whenever even the smallest speck of calculus (0.5 mm in diameter or less) is seen on the tooth surface there is a corresponding inflamed, bleeding and ulcerated site in the pocket lining exactly opposite that piece of calculus [2].

Nevertheless, closed scaling and root planing without endoscopy can give good short-term clinical results with shrinkage of probing depths and a decrease in gingival inflammation, but probing depths in deeper areas often slowly return [5]. A review of studies evaluating the effectiveness of various subgingival debridement procedures showed that 5–80% of treated roots harbor residual plaque or calculus, and the deeper the pockets and furcation involvements, the more deposits are left behind [7]. Up to 30% of the total surface area of treated roots may be covered with residual calculus, following subgingival scaling [7]. These deposits may serve as the basis for reinfection of the pocket.

Traditional blind scaling and root planing, especially if performed by inexperienced operators, can result in patient discomfort, unwarranted removal of cementum and dentin, and an increase in tooth sensitivity [8]. By contrast, a pilot study evaluating endoscopic subgingival scaling and root planing reported minimal negative sequela. The study also reported elimination of histologic signs of chronic inflammation at 6 months following a single course of endoscopic periodontal debridement. Also observed was bone repair and growth of a long junctional epithelium on previously diseased root surfaces [5].

In a large unpublished case series performed in the office of one of the authors, John Kwan, a retrospective analysis of patients who received endoscopic ultrasonic periodontal debridement was performed.

After routine periodontal examination, these patients were diagnosed with generalized and or localized moderate-to-advanced chronic inflammatory periodontal disease. When the patients were evaluated at 1 year or more following treatment, a dramatic reduction in probing depths was noted. The greatest improvement was noted on posterior teeth with initial deep pocket probing depths.

Study design

This was a nonblinded prospective outcomes study. Patients with moderate-to-advanced periodontal disease were examined and pocket probing depths were recorded in a computerized charting program. All probing measurements were performed using a manual periodontal probe. The examiner was calibrated for consistent recordings.

During the first 2 years' practicing with the periodontal endoscope (2002–2004), 270 consecutively treated patients were evaluated. All treated patients were given a course of systemic antibiotics; either metronidazole 500 mg bid × 7 days, or metronidazole and amoxicillin both 500 mg bid × 7 days, or azithromycin 500 mg qd × 3 days. Antibiotics were taken either before or immediately following treatment. All treatment was completed in one visit: full-mouth ultrasonic debridement with probing depths ≥4 mm endoscopically debrided.

Patients were seen for reevaluation and periodontal maintenance every 3 months, which included full-mouth periodontal charting, periodontal instrumentation, selective polish, and oral hygiene instruction. Final comparison probing was performed at 1 year or more.

71% reduced to 6–9 mm
20% reduced to ≤5 mm
n = 45 teeth

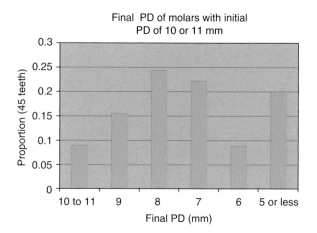

Final PD of molars with initial
PD of 10 or 11 mm

55% reduced to ≤5 mm
n = 284 teeth

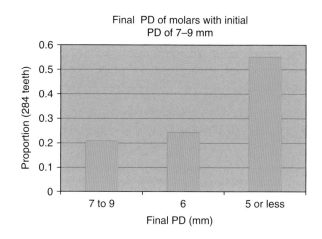

Final PD of molars with initial
PD of 7–9 mm

Starting at 5–6 mm:
69% reduced to ≤4 mm
n = 478 teeth

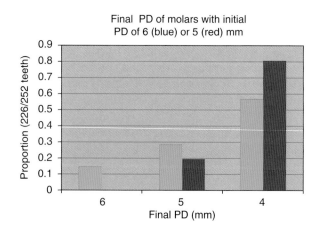

Final PD of molars with initial
PD of 6 (blue) or 5 (red) mm

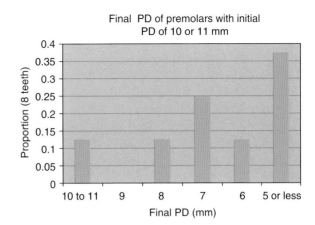

38% reduced to ≤5 mm
n = 8 teeth

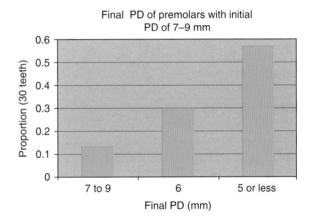

57% reduced to ≤5 mm
n = 30 teeth

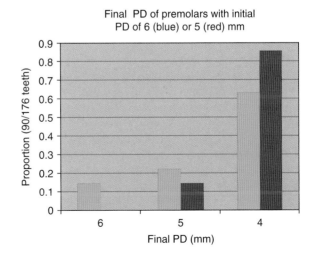

78% reduced to ≤4 mm
n = 266 teeth

71% reduced to ≤5 mm
n = 7 teeth

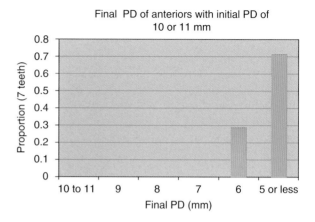

89% reduced to ≤5 mm
n = 57 teeth

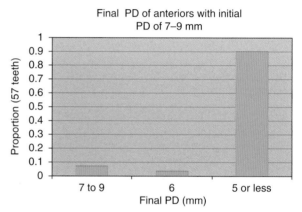

92% reduced to ≤4 mm
n = 246 teeth

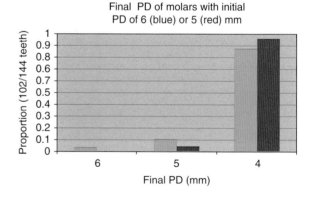

Conclusions

Reductions in probing depths were noted in all types of teeth, particularly in deeply pocketed posterior teeth. Proportionally, more teeth that began with deeper probing depths were reduced to ≤5mm PD at reevaluation. Ultrasonic endoscopic subgingival debridement in conjunction with systemic antibiotic

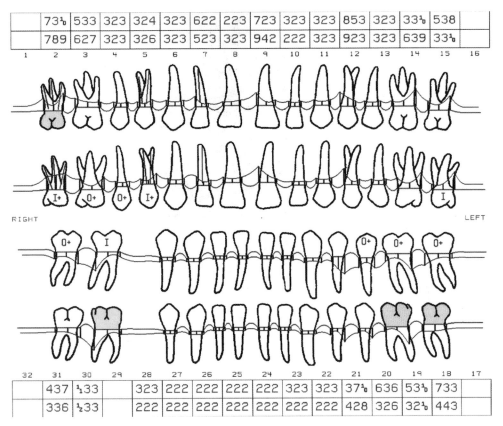

1	2	3	4	5	6	7	8	9	10	11	12	13	14	15	16
	73½	533	323	324	323	622	223	723	323	323	853	323	33½	538	
	789	627	323	326	323	523	323	942	222	323	923	323	639	33½	

RIGHT   LEFT

32	31	30	29	28	27	26	25	24	23	22	21	20	19	18	17
	437	½33		323	222	222	222	222	323	323	37½	636	53½	733	
	336	½33		222	222	222	222	222	222	222	428	326	32½	443	

Figure 3.11   Initial periodontal charting; pocket depths from 4 to 12 mm. Source: Reproduced with permission of John Y. Kwan, DDS.

uses reduced 7–9 mm PD in more than 50% of the teeth treated this way regardless of tooth type.

This subgingival microvisual debridement is a minimally invasive, nonsurgical option for patients with periodontal disease. The following is an example of a full-mouth ultrasonic dental endoscopic debridement treatment and follow-up (Figures 3.11, 3.12, 3.13, 3.14, 3.15, and 3.16).

Description of dental endoscopic technique

Periodontal endoscopy utilizes a two-handed technique: (i) the endoscope in the nondominant hand (similar to holding a dental mirror) and (ii) the powered instrument in the dominant hand, moving together around the tooth while cleaning. Rarely, a "view, instrument and view" technique is used when both the endoscope and explorer are unable to simultaneously access the area being scaled. Four explorer designs are used to visually access all surfaces of the teeth.

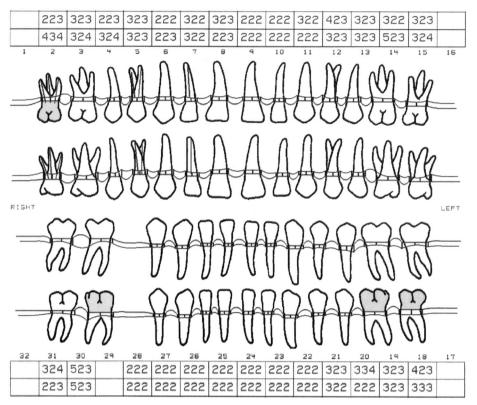

	2	3	4	5	6	7	8	9	10	11	12	13	14	15
	223	323	223	323	222	322	323	222	222	322	423	323	322	323
	434	324	324	323	223	322	223	222	222	222	323	323	523	324

RIGHT LEFT

32	31	30	29	28	27	26	25	24	23	22	21	20	19	18	17
	324	523		222	222	222	222	222	222	222	323	334	323	423	
	223	523		222	222	222	222	222	222	222	322	222	323	333	

Figure 3.12 Fifteen months post micro-ultrasonic endoscopic periodontal debridement, the deepest pockets now probe 4–5 mm. Source: Reproduced with permission of John Y. Kwan, DDS.

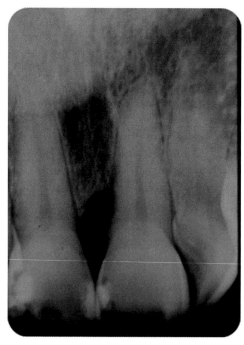

Figure 3.13 Pretreatment X-ray. Source: Reproduced with permission of John Y. Kwan, DDS.

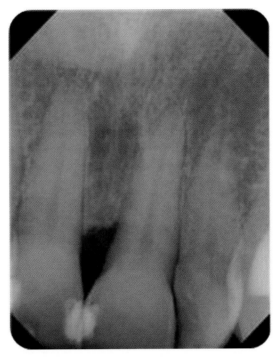

Figure 3.14   Fifteen months post treatment X-ray. Source: Reproduced with permission of John Y. Kwan, DDS.

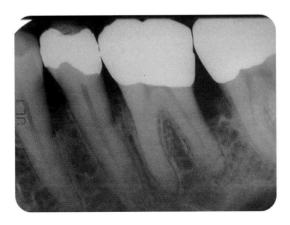

Figure 3.15   Pretreatment X-ray. Source: Reproduced with permission of John Y. Kwan, DDS.

It is the author's opinion that following a systematic approach, experienced dental endoscope clinicians may provide microvisual full-mouth debridement as quickly as, and possibly more efficiently than traditional periodontal debridement (Figure 3.17).

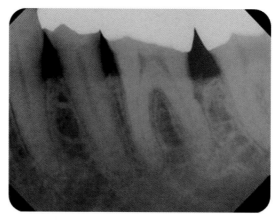

Figure 3.16 Fifteen months post-Tx X-ray. Source: Reproduced with permission of John Y. Kwan, DDS.

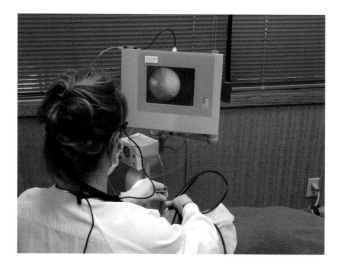

Figure 3.17 Two-handed dental endoscopy being performed. Source: Reproduced with permission of Perioscopy Incorporated.

Beginning and finishing with one explorer in each segment before starting with another explorer is an integral part of the systematic approach to endoscopic debridement. This method is similar to that taught for blind closed pocket instrumentation.

Ultrasonic powered instruments are the first choice for use with the periodontal endoscope. Typical ultrasonic inserts used are small and probe like. Endoscopically, they provide efficient root debridement, requiring only a small array of instruments. A full-mouth debridement typically requires only a straight probe-like universal ultrasonic tip with an occasional need for curved or angled tips. These nonbladed ultrasonic tips are also less likely to remove healthy root structure. Just

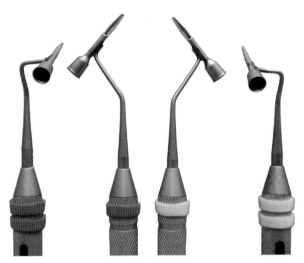

Figure 3.18   Dental endoscopy explorers: Right/right, right, left, left/left. Source: Reproduced with permission of Perioscopy Incorporated.

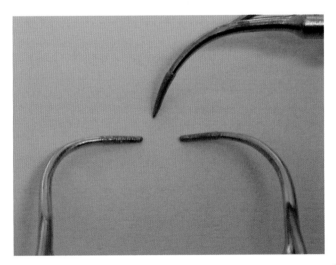

Figure 3.19   Magnetostrictive diamond-coated ultrasonic inserts. Source: Reproduced with permission of Perioscopy Incorporated.

as most providers develop preferences and proficiencies with certain instruments, their use with the dental endoscope should prove useful. Efficiency is enhanced by fewer instrument changes and more instrument adaptation (Figure 3.18).

Diamond-coated ultrasonic instruments are used for advanced instrumentation in the removal of rough (globular) cementum, tenacious calculus, overhanging restorations, and subgingival enamel anomalies. Because of their cutting power, advanced skill is required in the use of diamond-coated ultrasonic tips. This is not only true with the cutting function, but also to avoid damage to the explorer shield, sheath over the endoscope fiber, or the fiber itself (Figure 3.19).

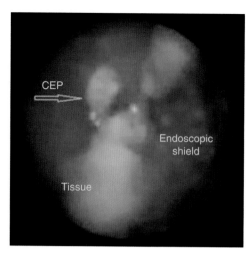

Figure 3.20 Grade I CEP.

Although bacterial plaque is the primary extrinsic etiologic factor for the initiation and progression of periodontal disease, anatomic factors such as cervical enamel projections (CEPs), enamel pearls, and developmental grooves are often associated with localized periodontal destruction because they may predispose the affected area to plaque accumulation, making personal oral hygiene and professional scaling more difficult, thereby increasing a patient's chance of periodontal breakdown. Enamel projections found in furcation areas of molars have been found to be highly susceptible to the creation of periodontal pockets because there is no connective tissue attachment to the enamel. As a result, a close association has been reported between enamel projections and furcation involvement [9,10].

Masters and Hoskins were the first to suggest the association of the CEP with periodontal disease and classified the projections into three grades based on the location of adjacent CEJs and furcations: Grade I indicates a short but distinct change in the contour of the CEJ extending toward the furcation, Grade II designates when the CEP approaches the furcation without making contact with it, and Grade III denotes that the CEP extends into the furcation.

Ectopic enamel removal is a common recommendation because it allows new attachment to form [9].

Figure 3.20 and corresponding video link available on the book companion website show cervical enamel projections found during endoscopic treatment on molar teeth that have developed periodontal infection. Using dental endoscopy, enamel projections may be removed quickly and efficiently in a minimally invasive, nonsurgical manner. Prior to dental endoscopy, these areas would have required surgical intervention to view and/or treat.

Grade l CEP appears as a small, flat projection that extends toward the furcation (Figure 3.20).

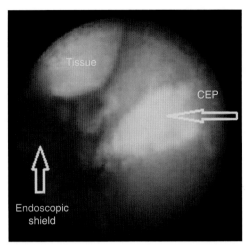

Figure 3.21   Grade II CEP.

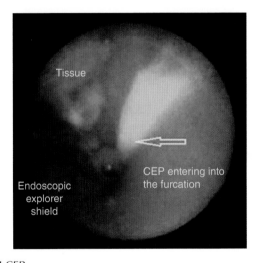

Figure 3.22   Grade III CEP.

Grade II CEP begins just under the CEJ and extends toward the entrance of the furcation, but does not enter. Depending on the size and thickness of an enamel projection, Grade-I and Grade-II CEPs may be removed with an ultrasonic insert on medium-to-high power using firm pressure; or if required, a more aggressive diamond-tipped insert may be used. It is recommended that these methods only be used with visualization because of their aggressive nature (Figure 3.21).

Figure 3.22 shows a Grade-III CEP entering into the furcation.

The video "Cervical enamel projections found in molar teeth with furcation involvement" is available on the book companion website.

Enamel pearls

Although bacterial plaque is a primary cause of the initiation and progression of periodontal disease, anatomic factors such as enamel pearls are often associated with advanced localized periodontal destruction [11]. Ectopic enamel removal is generally recommended during periodontal surgeries to allow new attachment to form [12]. With the advent of the dental endoscope, a diamond-tipped ultrasonic insert can remove enamel pearls nonsurgically. Figures 3.23 and 3.24 and corresponding video available on the book companion website show an endoscopic enameloplasty.

The video "enameloplasty visualized with the perioscope," is available on the book companion website.

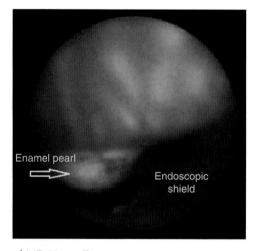

Figure 3.23   Enamel pearl MB #3 pre-Tx.

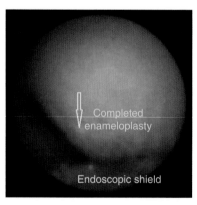

Figure 3.24   Post enameloplasty.

Dental endoscopic instruction

After training in the use of the dental endoscope, the initial learning curve typically takes about 10 patients. A practitioner usually enters the comfort zone after treating between 20 and 30 patients. Recommended training usually consists of an online video review, bench training, and patient hands-on training. This type of instruction is usually provided in-office and can also be provided as part of dental, dental hygiene, and periodontal clinical training (Figure 3.25).

Proper positioning of the patient is critical to allow for effective water evacuation. A low-volume suction device or saliva ejector, again properly positioned, is adequate to allow for treatment without an assistant. During treatment without the benefit of a mirror to retract, the sides of the endoscope explorer and ultrasonic instrument can be used to retract (tongue and cheek).

Instruments are positioned looking in the mouth, and then the operator focuses on the screen to govern movements. Medium-to-medium plus power is used with ultrasonic instrumentation, using lateral pressure for more power (which is contrary to most teaching, but the benefit is very evident when cleaning endoscopically). The more tenacious the deposit, the more amplitude or power is used, utilizing smaller movements over deposits until the area is completely clean (Figure 3.26).

Subgingival visualization has shown that instrument access is far more predictable and efficient when the root surface and instrument can be simultaneously viewed.

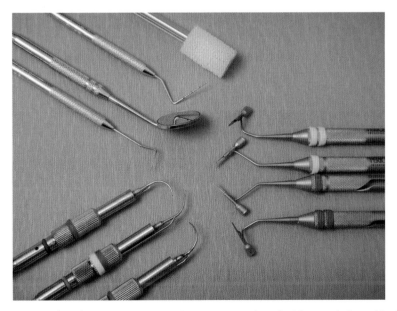

Figure 3.25   Dental endoscopic tray setup. Source: Reproduced with permission of Perioscopy Incorporated.

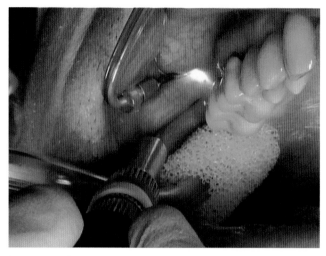

Figure 3.26   Endoscope explorer and ultrasonic instrument retracting the cheek. Source: Reproduced with permission of Perioscopy Incorporated.

Decisions in selecting nonsurgical endoscopic treatment

When initiating any nonsurgical periodontal therapy, clinicians must be aware of the following aspects:

- the objective of treatment;
- limitations of treatment (i.e., tooth anatomy, pocket depth, and operator error);
- whether treatment recommendations are in line with the severity of the disease.

Objectives of treatment include

- ameliorating or arrest the disease process;
- attempting to maintain or possibly regenerate periodontal/peri-implant support;
- reducing the periodontal/peri-implant inflammatory process.

Peri-implant diseases present in two forms: (i) peri-implant mucositis and (ii) peri-implantitis. Both are characterized by an inflammatory reaction in the tissues surrounding an implant [13]. It is accepted by some that peri-implant mucositis is the precursor of peri-implantitis, as it is accepted that gingivitis is the precursor of periodontitis. However, similar to the causal relationship between gingivitis and periodontitis, peri-implant mucositis does not necessarily progress to peri-implantitis [14].

Prevalence of peri-implantitis has been widely reported [15]. Peri-implantitis has been characterized by some as an inflammatory process around an implant, which includes both soft tissue inflammation and progressive loss of supporting bone beyond biological bone remodeling [13]. Some believe that peri-implantitis, like periodontitis, occurs primarily as a result of an overwhelming bacterial insult and subsequent host immune response. For this group, the primary objective for treating peri-implantitis is similar to that for treating peri-implant mucositis, which is the elimination of the biofilm from the implant surface [14].

Although sharing similarities with periodontitis in both the bacterial initiators and key immune components to those insults, the rate of disease progression and the severity of inflammatory signs for peri-implantitis may be different [14]. The microbiology of peri-implantitis is more diverse than that of periodontitis [16]. Histologically, peri-implantitis is much more infiltrative near the alveolar crest and often lacks a protective layer of tissue over the bone as we typically see in periodontitis [17,18].

Data has shown that peri-implant infections are often responsible for late failures [19]. Treatment of peri-implant disease may be found in Chapter 5.

Peri-implantitis is an infection of the tissue around an implant, resulting in the loss of supporting bone. Risk factors for peri-implantitis consist of a history of periodontitis, dental plaque, poor oral hygiene, smoking, alcohol consumption, and diabetes. A clinical diagnosis indicates inflammatory signs including bleeding on probing with or without suppuration and a peri-implant pocket depth of ≥5 mm [20]. Aggressive treatment of the underlying cause of these negative clinical findings is indicated when this diagnosis is made. The endoscope is extremely valuable in both the diagnosis and treatment of peri-implantitis and should be employed as soon as feasible on these individuals.

Endoscopic examination for patients with peri-implant diseases often reveals foreign material attached to the implant surface or to the prosthetic superstructure. White highly reflective material is often seen attached to the implant or its superstructure. The best evidence available at this time indicates that this material may be dental cement.

Utilizing the periodontal endoscope, subgingival residual cement associated with peri-implant disease may be diagnosed and removed. Endoscopically, cement removal may be accomplished utilizing either ultrasonic and or hand instruments.

Although dental endoscopy affords clinicians the opportunity to provide meticulous instrumentation, appropriate treatment recommendations should be based on the level of disease to be treated and operator experience (Figure 3.27).

Areas where periodontal endoscopic debridement is difficult include

- very inflamed pockets;
- abscesses;
- distal furcations of maxillary molars;
- narrow furcations and class III furcations;
- curved roots;
- close root proximity;
- grossly overcontoured restorations.

Although mechanical debridement is essential in removing the bacterial bioburden from root surfaces in nonsurgical periodontal therapy, endoscopic debridement may also incorporate adjuncts. These are the same adjuncts that many clinicians use with closed and open debridement, and these may include

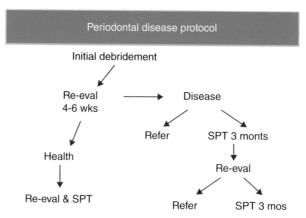

Figure 3.27 Periodontal disease treatment protocol.

systemic antibiotics, low-dose doxycycline hyclate 20 mg, local delivery antibiotics such as 1.0 mg minocycline HCl, biologics such as enamel matrix derivatives, or rhPDGF, dental lasers for nonsurgical sulcular debridement (sometimes referred to as laser curettage, pocket sterilization, or laser pocket disinfection) and various chemical disinfection options.

In the opinion of the authors, actively progressing periodontitis is almost always associated with specific bacterial infections and may require the adjunctive use of systemic antibiotic therapy. By entering periodontal tissues and the periodontal pocket via serum, systemic antibiotics can affect organisms outside the reach of instruments, or topical anti-infective chemotherapeutics. Systemic antibiotic therapy also has the potential to suppress periodontal pathogens residing on the tongue or other oral surfaces, thereby delaying subgingival recolonization of pathogens [21]. Since periodontal lesions often harbor a mixture of pathogenic bacteria, drug combination therapies have gained increasing importance and may even be required for eradication and prevention of periodontal infections by known periodontal pathogens that invade subepithelial periodontal tissue or colonize extradental domains from which they may translocate to periodontal sites [21]. Many clinicians prescribe antibiotics empirically, based on clinical experience and/or the patient's medical history and sensitivity to the desired antibiotics. The rationale supporting this approach is that most pathogens are susceptible to the same antibiotics, and identification of specific bacteria is reserved for those situations where there is no or minimal clinical improvement after a course of systemic antibiotics or to ensure the elimination of the target bacteria [22].

Adjunctive antimicrobial agents such as systemic antibiotics, locally delivered antibiotics, and antimicrobial irrigation have been shown to improve treatment outcomes in patients presenting with destructive periodontal disease [23].

The following cases utilize varying adjuncts, but the emphasis and commonality is the ability to endoscopically visualize and thoroughly debride diseased root surfaces.

The following example case reports demonstrate positive clinical and radiographic healing when thorough root debridement is accomplished through minimally invasive endoscopic debridement.

Case 1—Robert Gottlieb, DDS, and Suzanne Newkirk, RDH, Richland, WA

This 47-year-old female had a history of yearly cleanings, orthognathic surgery, orthodontics, and gingival tissue grafting in the mandibular anterior teeth. She was referred for periodontal evaluation and for upper left and lower left discomfort. Clinical and radiographic examination revealed periodontal probing depths of 4–5mm, bleeding on probing, and a significant amount of calculus throughout her mouth.

The patient presented with a class III bilateral Angles classification, with signs and symptoms of bruxism and an anterior open bite. A diagnosis of the American Academy of Periodontology (AAP) case type II–III (early-to-moderate) periodontal disease was made (Figures 3.28, 3.29, 3.30, and 3.31).

A nonsurgical treatment plan was developed consisting of ultrasonic endoscopic debridement that was completed in two appointments. Post-treatment instructions were provided to the patient for the care of her mouth post-endoscopic debridement, and the patient was scheduled for reevaluation 8 weeks post treatment to assess tissue response of endoscopic therapy. Periodontal recharting was performed indicating that healing had taken place, and the patient was scheduled for periodontal maintenance every 3 months to include periodontal charting, instrumentation, and polish.

Two years post endoscopic debridement, the patient has remained stable and is maintaining a favorable clinical outcome with an overall improved dentition and probing depths no greater than 3mm (Figure 3.32, 3.33, 3.34).

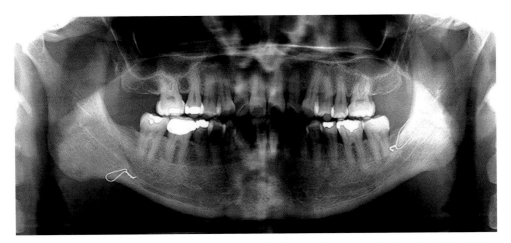

Figure 3.28   Pretreatment panographic radiograph. Source: Courtesy of Robert Gottlieb, DDS and Suzanne Newkirk, RDH.

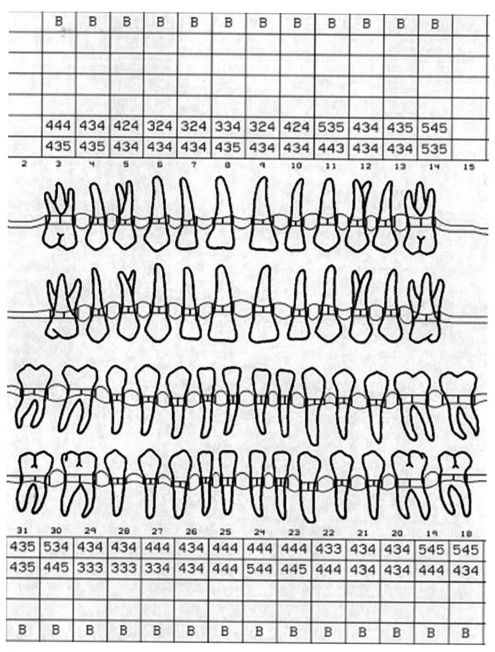

	B	B	B	B	B	B	B	B	B	B	B	B	
	444	434	424	324	324	334	324	424	535	434	435	545	
	435	435	434	434	434	435	434	434	443	434	434	535	
2	3	4	5	6	7	8	9	10	11	12	13	14	15

31	30	29	28	27	26	25	24	23	22	21	20	19	18
435	534	434	434	444	434	444	444	444	433	434	434	545	545
435	445	333	333	334	434	444	544	445	444	434	434	444	434
B	B	B	B	B	B	B	B	B	B	B	B	B	B

Figure 3.29 Pre-Tx periodontal charting. Source: Courtesy of Robert Gottlieb, DDS and Suzanne Newkirk, RDH.

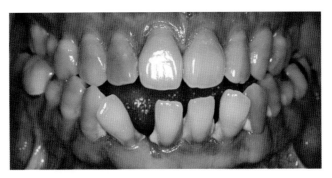

Figure 3.30   Pre-Tx photo facials. Source: Courtesy of Robert Gottlieb, DDS and Suzanne Newkirk, RDH.

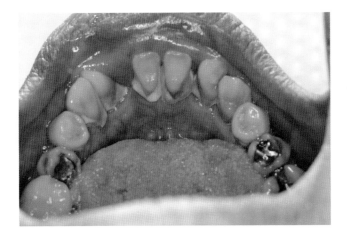

Figure 3.31   Pre-Tx photo mandibular d lingual. Source: Courtesy of Robert Gottlieb, DDS and Suzanne Newkirk, RDH.

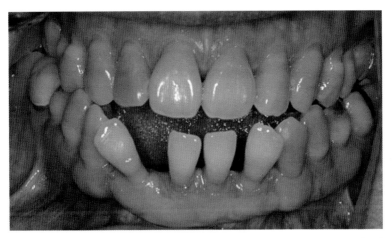

Figure 3.32   Post-Tx photo, facials 9 months' post treatment. Source: Courtesy of Robert Gottlieb, DDS and Suzanne Newkirk, RDH.

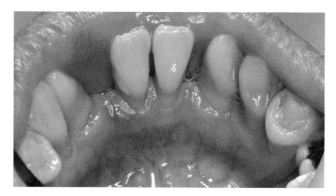

Figure 3.33 Nine months post-Tx mandibular linguals. Source: Courtesy of Robert Gottlieb, DDS and Suzanne Newkirk, RDH.

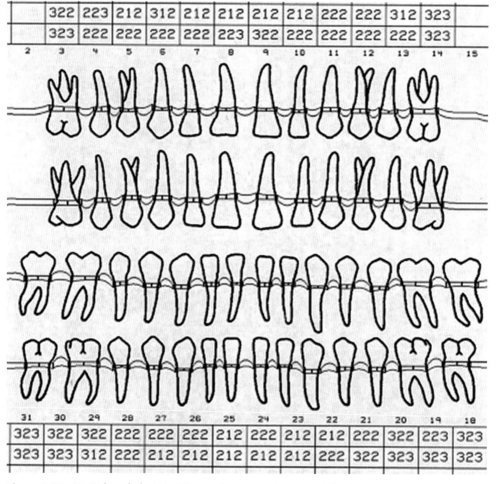

Figure 3.34 Periodontal charting 30 months post endoscopic debridement. Source: Courtesy of Robert Gottlieb, DDS and Suzanne Newkirk, RDH.

Case 2—David Trylovich, DDS, MS, and Shelly Andreoli, RDH, Las Vegas, NV

This 67-year-old male patient had been consulting his general dentist for 20 years prior to being referred to a periodontist for periodontal evaluation. The referring dentist expected extraction of #26 and implant placement into the edentulous area.

Clinical and radiographic examination revealed a periodontal probing depth of 12 mm on the distal surface of #26 with associated bleeding on probing, Class I mobility on the Miller scale on #25 and Class II mobility on #26. Localized recession of 1–2 mm was present in the lower anterior teeth.

A diagnosis of localized AAP case type IV (advanced or severe) periodontal disease was made (Figure 3.35 and 3.36).

Full-mouth nonsurgical endoscopic debridement was provided under local anesthesia and completed in three visits. In addition, application of 1.0 mg minocycline HCl was provided subgingivally to the distal surface on #26. A prescription for doxycycline hyclate 20 mg was given to the patient to take two times per day for 90 days.

Eight weeks post periodontal treatment, the patient returned for reevaluation to assess tissue response. Full-mouth periodontal charting was performed; periodontal maintenance and an additional application of 1.0 mg minocycline HCl was placed subgingivally into the distal surface of #26 (Figure 3.37 and 3.38).

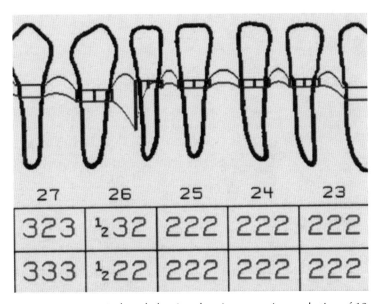

Figure 3.35   Pre-treatment periodontal charting showing extensive pocketing of 12 mm. Source: Courtesy of David Trylovich, DDS, MS and Shelly Andreoli, RDH.

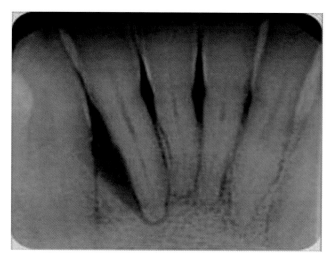

Figure 3.36 Pre-Tx radiograph showing bone loss to the apex on the distal of #26. Source: Courtesy of David Trylovich, DDS, MS and Shelly Andreoli, RDH.

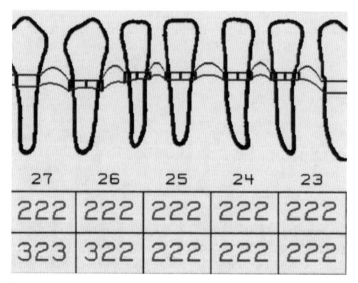

Figure 3.37 Three years post dental endoscopic treatment and placement of minocycline HCl, probing depths have reduced dramatically. Source: Courtesy of David Trylovich, DDS, MS and Shelly Andreoli, RDH.

Eight years post endoscopic debridement and application of locally applied minocycline, the patient is maintaining a favorable clinical outcome with an overall improved dentition; #26 shows decreased pocketing from 12 to 2 mm and radiographic bone repair.

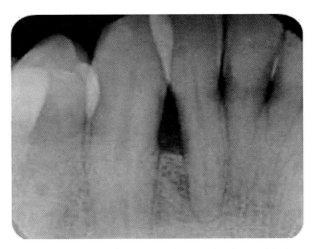

Figure 3.38   The post treatment X-ray showing evidence of radiographic bone repair. Source: Courtesy of David Trylovich, DDS, MS and Shelly Andreoli, RDH.

Case 3—Richard Longbottom, DDS, and Wendy Williams, RDH, Auckland, NZ

This 62-year-old Asian Female had no history of previous periodontal treatment and received twice-yearly cleanings provided by her general practioner. The patient lost the maxillary left second molar (#15) and was referred to the periodontist for periodontal evaluation.

A comprehensive periodontal evaluation revealed probing depths of 4–10mm, with generalized bleeding on probing, localized gingival recession of 1–3mm was noted throughout the dentition, and a generalized AAP case type III–IV (moderate-to-severe) periodontal diagnosis was made.

Because of financial constraints, a nonsurgical treatment plan was developed, consisting of ultrasonic scaling under local anesthetic, which was as completed in two visits. In addition, amoxicillin 500mg and metronidazole 400mg, both three times a day for 6 days was prescribed concurrent with initial therapy. Fourteen months later, the patient underwent ultrasonic endoscopic debridement, which was completed in two visits under local anesthesia. Povidone-iodine was irrigated into the periodontal pockets (Figure 3.39 and 3.40).

A periapical (PA) radiograph was taken of #30 (first image), and a probing depth of 10mm was recorded on the distal buccal surface of #30. Three months post endoscopic debridement, periodontal maintenance was provided, which included full-mouth periodontal charting, instrumentation, and polish. Another PA radiograph of #30 was taken and a probing depth of 5mm was recorded on the distal buccal surface of #30 (Figure 3.41 and 3.42).

Twenty-four months post endoscopic debridement, the final periapical radiograph was taken (see Figure 3.41) and a probing depth of 2mm was recorded on

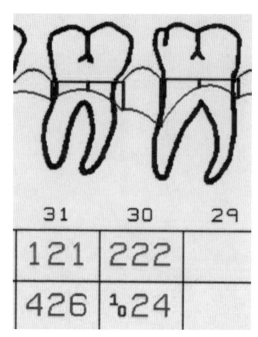

31	30	29
121	222	
426	¹₀24	

Figure 3.39 Pretreatment periodontal charting. Source: Courtesy of Richard Longbottom, DDS and Wendy Williams, RDH.

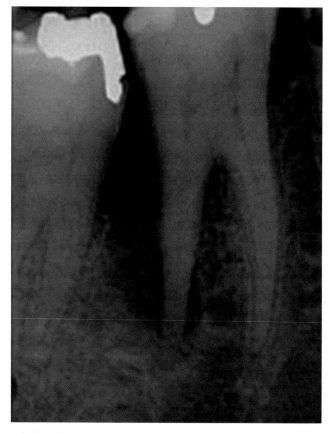

Figure 3.40 Radiograph showing a 10 mm pocket on the DB #30 and associated radiographic bone loss. Source: Courtesy of Richard Longbottom, DDS and Wendy Williams, RDH.

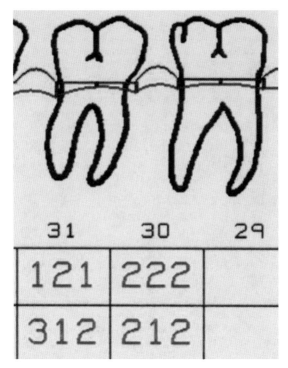

31	30	29
121	222	
312	212	

Figure 3.41 Periodontal charting. Source: Courtesy of Richard Longbottom, DDS and Wendy Williams, RDH.

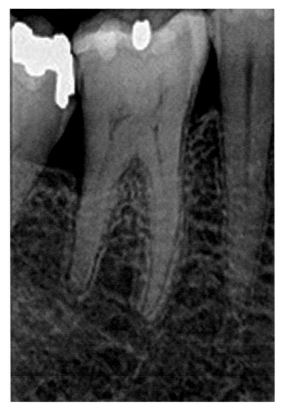

Figure 3.42 Radiograph 24 months post treatment. Source: Courtesy of Richard Longbottom, DDS and Wendy Williams, RDH.

the distal buccal surface of #30. The patient has maintained a 3-month periodontal maintenance schedule. Periodontal indicates a reduction in pocket depths and #30 shows evidence of radiographic bone repair.

Case 4—Dr Robert Gottlieb and Suzanne Newkirk, RDH, Richland, WA

This 59-year-old patient received twice-yearly cleanings by her general practioner, and no history of previous periodontal treatment. Her chief complaint was that her fixed partial denture (#'s 9–11) "keeps losing gum tissue," and the patient "felt it was ugly." This was the third fixed partial denture that had been placed. A comprehensive periodontal examination revealed periodontal probing depths of 4–9 mm, with associated generalized bleeding on probing. Localized Class I mobility and gingival recession of 1–3 mm was noted throughout the dentition. Radiographic bone loss around the fixed partial denture was noted, and a diagnosis of AAP case type III–IV (moderate-to -severe) periodontal disease was made (Figure 3.43, 3.44, and 3.45).

The patient was initially recommended full-mouth laser surgery (Laser-assisted new attachment 0rocedure), implant placement in the edentulous area #10 and crown lengthening, but the patient declined all surgical options. A nonsurgical treatment plan of ultrasonic endoscopic debridement was made, and the patient was prescribed azithromycin (250 mg × 6), two to be taken the day of treatment, and then one per day until gone. Endoscopic debridement with adjunctive nonsurgical laser pocket disinfection was completed in two visits under local anesthesia. Periodontal maintenance was provided every 3 months to include full-mouth periodontal charting, instrumentation, and polish. The replacement of #'s 7–9 fixed partial denture was coordinated with the referring general dentist (Figure 3.46, 3.47, 3.48, 3.49, and 3.50)

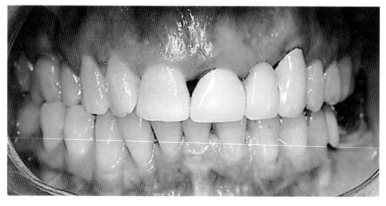

Figure 3.43 Pre-Tx photo, upper anterior bridge. Source: Courtesy of Dr. Robert Gottlieb and Suzanne Newkirk, RDH.

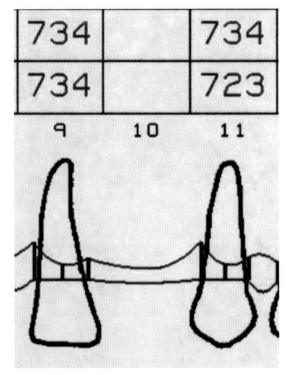

Figure 3.44   Pre-Tx perio charting. Source: Courtesy of Dr. Robert Gottlieb and Suzanne Newkirk, RDH.

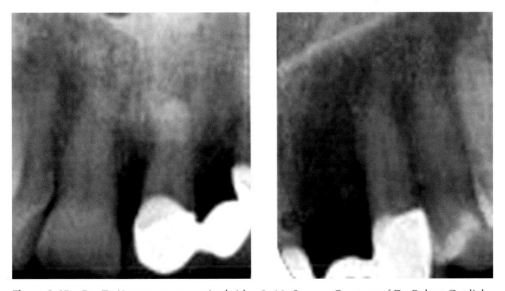

Figure 3.45   Pre-Tx X-rays upper anterior bridge 9–11. Source: Courtesy of Dr. Robert Gottlieb and Suzanne Newkirk, RDH.

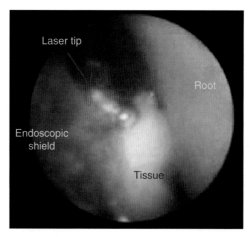

Figure 3.46 Laser tip viewed using the dental endoscope. Source: Courtesy of Dr. Robert Gottlieb and Suzanne Newkirk, RDH.

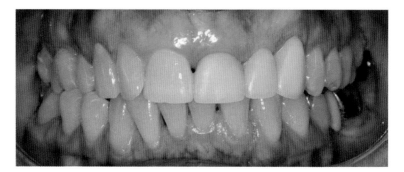

Figure 3.47 Post restorative bridge upper anterior 9–11. Source: Courtesy of Dr. Robert Gottlieb and Suzanne Newkirk, RDH.

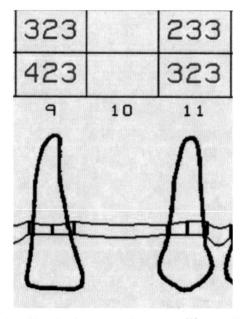

Figure 3.48 Periodontal probing depths 15 months post endoscopic debridement. Source: Courtesy of Dr. Robert Gottlieb and Suzanne Newkirk, RDH.

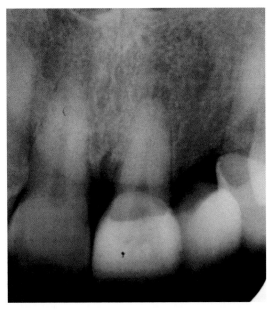

Figure 3.49 Radiograph of upper anterior bridge 3 years post endoscopic debridement. Source: Courtesy of Dr. Robert Gottlieb and Suzanne Newkirk, RDH.

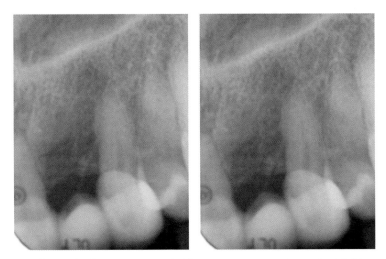

Figure 3.50 Radiograph of upper anterior bridge 3 years post endoscopic debridement. Source: Courtesy of Dr. Robert Gottlieb and Suzanne Newkirk, RDH.

Three years post ultrasonic endoscopic debridement, the patient is maintaining a generalized favorable clinical outcome. Periodontal charting reveals overall improvement with generalized decreased probing depths, and radiographic bone repair is evident on the fixed partial denture abutments.

As the above case reports demonstrate, meticulous instrumentation provided by dental endoscopic treatment can render superior clinical outcomes. Clinicians have discovered the benefits of this technology and are providing nonsurgical endoscopic diagnosis and treatment in all parts of the world and using varied approaches to therapy.

Summary

Ultrasonic endoscopic periodontal debridement is a minimally invasive microvisual technology utilized for the nonsurgical treatment of periodontal disease. The dental endoscope is also a valuable diagnostic tool for evaluation of caries, root fractures, root resorption/perforations, residual cement around teeth and implant restorations, and subgingival anomalies. As with any advanced dental instrumentation and skill, this technology requires focused attention, a desire to learn, training, practice, and patience. This skill set combined with the microvisual capacity of dental and periodontal endoscopy is providing dentistry, dental hygiene, and periodontics with a valuable and very different "vision" toward dental and periodontal health.

References

1. Geibel, M.-A. (2006) Development of a new micro-endoscope for odontological application. *European Journal of Medical Research*, **11**, 123–127.
2. Pattison, A.M. & Pattison, G.L. (2003) Dimensions of dental hygiene, periodontal instrumentation transformed. *Dimensions of Dental Hygiene*, **1 (2)**, 18–20, 22.
3. Wilson, T.G. Jr., Harrel, S.K., Nunn, M.E., Francis, B. & Webb, K. (2008) The relationship between the presence of tooth-borne subgingival deposits and inflammation found with a dental endoscope. *Journal of Periodontology*, **79 (11)**, 2029–2035.
4. Caffesse, R.G., Sweeney, P.L. & Smith, B.A. (1986) Scaling and root planing with and without periodontal flap surgery. *Journal of Clinical Periodontology*, **13**, 205–210.
5. Wilson, T.G. Jr., Carnio, J., Schenk, R. & Myers, G. (2008) Absence of histologic signs of chronic inflammation following closed subgingival scaling and root planing using the dental endoscope: Human biopsies—A pilot study. *Journal of Periodontology*, **79 (11)**, 2036–2041.
6. Rabbani, G.M., Ash, M.M. Jr. & Caffesse, R.G. (1981) The effectiveness of subgingival scaling and root planing in calculus removal. *Journal of Periodontology*, **52**, 119–123.
7. Petersilka, G.J., Ehmke, B. & Flemming, T.F. (2002) Antimicrobial effects of mechanical debridement. *Periodontal 2000*, **28**, 56–71.
8. Slots, J. (2012) Low-cost periodontal therapy. *Periodontol 2000*, **60 (1)**, 110–137.
9. Gorthi, C., Reddy, V. & Rani, K.R. Significance of cervical enamel projections in periodontal treatment. *Indian Journal of Dental Advancements*, **2 (4)**, 352–355.
10. Romeo, U., Palaia, G., Botti, R., Nardi, A., Del Vecchio, A., Tenore, G. & Polimeni, A. (2011) Enamel pearls as a predisposing factor to localized periodontitis. *Quintessence International*, **42 (1)**, 69–71.
11. Alizadeh Tabari, Z., Kadkhodazadeh, M. & Khademi, M. (2011) Enamel pearl as a predisposing factor to localized severe attachment loss: a case report. *Research Journal of Medical Sciences*, **5 (3)**, 141–144.

12. Goldstein, A.R. (1979) Enamel pearls as contributing factor in periodontal breakdown. *Journal of the American Dental Association*, **99 (2)**, 210–211.
13. Sanz, M. & Chapple, I.L. (2012) Clinical research on peri-implant diseases: Consensus report of Working Group 4. *Journal of Clinical Periodontology*, **39 (Suppl. 12)**, 202–206.
14. Rosen, P., Clem D., Cochran, D., Froum, S., McAllister, B., Renvert, S. & Wang, H.L. (2013) Peri-implant mucositis and peri-implantitis. *Journal of Periodontology*, **84 (4)**, 436–443. doi: 10.1902/jop.2013.134001
15. Zitzmann, N.U. & Berglundh, T. (2008) Definition and prevalence of peri-implant diseases. *Journal of Clinical Periodontology*, **35 (Suppl. 8)**, 286–291.
16. Koyanagi, T., Sakamoto, M., Takeuchi, Y., Maruyama, N., Ohkuma, M. & Izumi, Y. (2013) Comprehensive microbiological findings in periimplantitis and periodontitis. *Journal of Clinical Periodontology*, **40 (3)**, 218–226.
17. Berglundh, T., Zitzmann, N.U. & Donati, M. (2011) Are peri-implantitis lesions different from periodontitis lesions? *Journal of Clinical Periodontology*, **38 (Suppl. 11)**, 188–202.
18. Lang, N.P., Berglundh, T. on Behalf of Working Group 4 of the Seventh European Workshop on Periodontology (2011) Periimplant diseases: Where are we now?— Consensus of the Seventh European Workshop on Periodontology. *Journal of Clinical Periodontology*, **38 (Suppl. 11)**, 178–181.
19. Sakka, S. & Coulthard, P. (2011) Implant failure: Etiology and complications. *Medicina Oral Patologia Oral y Cirugia Bucal*, **16 (1)**, e42–e44.
20. Nguyen-Hieu, T., Borghetti, A. & Aboudharam, G. (2012) Peri-implantitis: From diagnosis to therapeutics. *Journal of Investigative and Clinical Dentistry*, **3 (2)**, 79–94.
21. Slots, J. & Ting, M.M. (2002) Systemic antibiotics in the treatment of periodontal disease. *Periodontal 2000*, **28**, 106–176.
22. Serio, F.G. & Serio, C.L. (2006) Systemic and local antibiotics and host modulation in periodontal therapy: Where are we now? Part I. *Inside Dentistry*, **2 (2)**.
23. Slots, J. (2002) Selection of antimicrobial agents in periodontal therapy. *Journal of Periodontal Research*, **37**, 389–398.

4 Endoscope Use in Daily Hygiene Practice

Kara Webb and Angela R. Anderson

The images in this section are to be used to provide orientation before accessing the video link (available on the book companion website). Figure 4.1 shows the clinical representation of how the endoscope shield is placed in the sulcus. The remaining images are representative of the subgingival environment.

In the past, dental hygienists had traditional closed subgingival scaling and root planing as the only option for treating periodontal disease. Technology brought hygiene to the next level with the introduction of dental endoscopy over a decade ago. It has become an invaluable tool for the hygienist in the treatment of periodontal disease and peri-implantitis. The endoscope aids in diagnosis and improves scaling outcomes. Learning to use the endoscope takes time; but with patience and determination, hygienists will wonder how they practiced without it.

Advantages

The endoscope provides advantages for the patient as well as the hygienist. It offers a way to remove calculus to a degree that prior to its introduction was only possible with periodontal flap surgery. We are able to treat the disease early and to obtain a more thorough, complete scaling in a closed environment often saving the patient the pain and discomfort of a surgical procedure. Calculus is often difficult to remove; therefore, visualization helps the clinician know when

Minimally Invasive Periodontal Therapy: Clinical Techniques and Visualization Technology, First Edition.
Edited by Stephen K. Harrel and Thomas G. Wilson Jr.
© 2015 John Wiley & Sons, Inc. Published 2015 by John Wiley & Sons, Inc.
Companion Website: www.wiley.com/go/harrel/minimallyinvasive

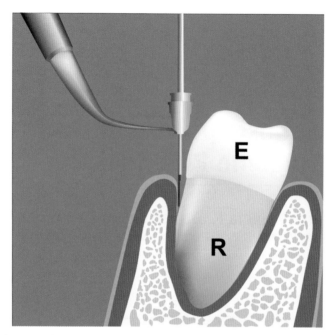

Figure 4.1   Endoscope shown placed in the sulcus at the level of the CEJ.

the deposits have been completely removed without unnecessarily removing additional tooth structure. For the first time, the endoscope allows the hygienist to see how the instrument adapts to the tooth surface in the sulcus. Watching this process as it happens allows the hygienist to see how to best adapt the instrument around line angles, furcations, and other difficult areas to clean, thereby helping to refine scaling techniques benefiting the hygienist when working without the endoscope.

Learning curve

There are two aspects to the learning curve of using the endoscope. The first is recognizing what is in the field of vision (Figure 4.2). Learning to identify the common landmarks (the CEJ, furcations, restorative margins, etc.) and pathology (caries, cracks, deposits, etc., Figures 4.2, 4.3, 4.4, 4.5, 4.6, 4.7, and 4.8) happens in a short time period. The second is learning to work with the instrument. There are two different approaches for using instruments to remove subgingival deposits. One approach places the endoscope into the sulcus for initial visualization to locate and identify the type of deposit. The endoscope is removed and scaling takes place. The endoscope is then placed back into the sulcus to view the tooth surface and evaluate the efficacy of scaling. With this technique, it usually takes several cycles to achieve the end result. A second approach, where there is adequate room, uses both hands: one for the endoscope and the other for the scaling instruments. This involves training the nondominant hand and has the longest learning curve.

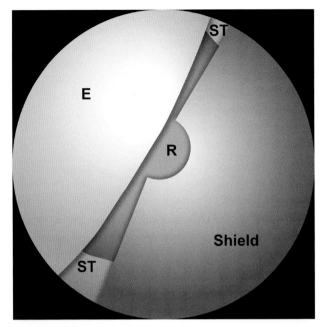

Figure 4.2   Endoscopic view of a healthy sulcus with enamel (E) and root surface (R) on the left and the endoscope shield on the right. Soft tissue (ST) is located between the tooth and the endoscope and is pink in color, indicating health.

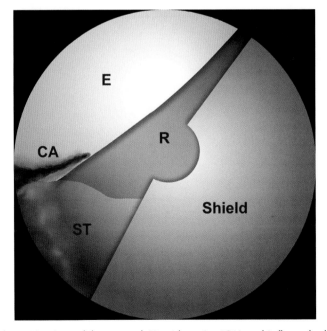

Figure 4.3   Endoscopic view of the enamel (E) with caries (CA) and inflamed adjacent soft tissue (ST) on the left. The root surface (R) is also visible between the endoscope shield and the enamel. The endoscope shield is on the right.

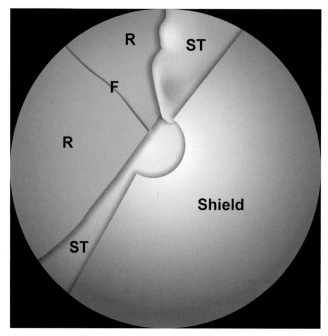

Figure 4.4   Root surface (R) of a tooth with a vertical fracture (F). The endoscope shield (S) is on the right. Soft tissue (ST) is in between the root and the shield.

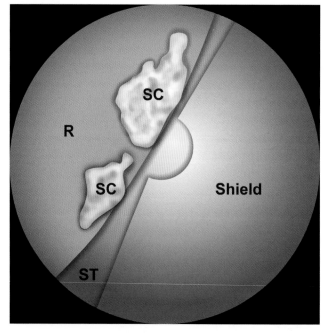

Figure 4.5   Black subgingival calculus (SC) which refracts yellow when viewed by the endoscope is present on the root surface (R). The endoscope shield is on the right. Soft tissue (ST) is in between the root and the shield.

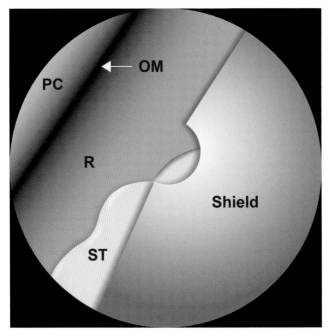

Figure 4.6   Open margin (OM) between the porcelain crown (PC) and the root surface (R). The endoscope shield is on the right. Soft tissue (ST) is in the lower left of the image.

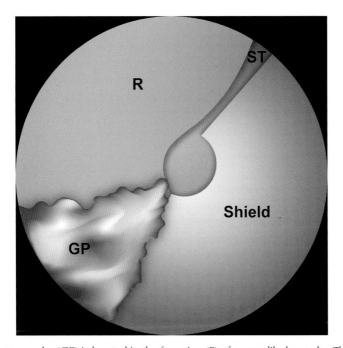

Figure 4.7   Gutta percha (GP) is located in the furcation (F) of a mandibular molar. The gutta percha shows up light pink to beige on the bottom left of the image. The endoscope shield is on the right.

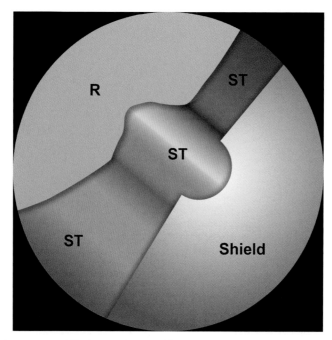

Figure 4.8   Soft tissue (ST) fills the void created by resorption (RP). The endoscope shield is on the right. The root surface (R) is on the left.

Anesthetic-local versus subgingival topical anesthetic

The discomfort level of the patient depends on the depth of the pocket and root sensitivity. In areas where the pocket is 5 mm or less and there is no dentinal sensitivity, topical anesthetics that can be applied directly into the sulcus work well. Local anesthesia is recommended in areas where the pocket depth is greater than 5 mm or the patient has thermal sensitivity.

Diagnostic

In a dental practice, there are often situations where a patient presents with an infection around a tooth; and after clinical examination and radiographs, the cause of the infection is still undetermined. The dental endoscope can be used to visualize the subgingival area to see if the cause is apparent. Root fractures, endodontic perforations, subgingival caries, root resorption, and crown margin discrepancies are some common issues (Figures 4.2, 4.3, 4.4, 4.5, 4.6, 4.7, and 4.8).

Increase in pocket probing depth

Traditional scaling with hand instrumentation and power scalers often leave burnished deposits behind that continue to cause irritation to the soft tissue. Increase in pocket depth and bleeding on probing are primarily due to this residual subgingival calculus. Periodontal maintenance patients that have been stable but begin to show a localized increase in probing depth that remains after maintenance can benefit from this procedure.

Chronic unacceptable probing depths are often found in areas of complex root anatomy such as developmental grooves, furcations, and enamel projections. When these anatomical features are present, it is often difficult to know when the area is free from deposits because the grooves become full and the calculus becomes smooth from repeated scaling. Working with the endoscope has proven that a smooth surface does not necessarily mean clean. The use of the endoscope gives the benefit of magnified sight in addition to tactile sensitivity.

Traditional scalers and ultrasonics can be used with the endoscope. It can also be helpful to have additional instruments such as diamond-coated files, mini after fives scalers, files, and ultrathin piezo tips. Piezo scalers have more control options and thinner tips.

Implants

The dental implant that has inflammation in the surrounding tissue and often an increase in pocket probing depth frequently has excess cement from the restorative process (Figure 4.9a and b). In the process of removal, the cement often breaks up into small pieces that become imbedded into the surrounding soft tissue. The endoscope allows the clinician to see where the cement is located and after scaling to see if there is any residual cement in the soft tissue that would need curettage.

One approach suggests only using graphite or titanium instruments on implants, but cement by nature is tenacious and is not removed easily. Most often traditional instruments are needed to remove the cement. Cement is most often located around the collar of the implant; and therefore, scaling with traditional instruments does not damage the main body of the implant.

Limitations

The endoscope does not come without limitations. The clinician must consider root morphology and severity of inflammation. The complexity of multirooted teeth makes it difficult to see the entire root surface and access every curve and indentation. Roots can be close together creating a furcation that is narrow and inaccessible with the tip of the endoscope or scaling instrument.

If the tissue has severe inflammation, it can completely block the view of the fiber-optic tip of the endoscope. The tissue folds around the shield, which holds the fiber optic, obstructing the view. Bleeding can also block the view of the tooth surface. When the disease is generalized, most clinicians experienced in endoscopy find it helpful to do closed subgingival scaling and root planing a few weeks prior to the use of the endoscope to minimize inflammation and bleeding, therefore optimizing the field of vision.

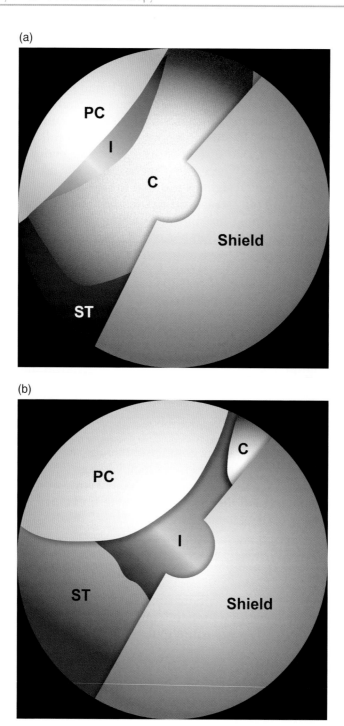

Figure 4.9 Implant (I) with residual cement (C). In (a), part of the implant can be seen between the porcelain crown (PC) and the cement (C). Inflammation of the soft tissue (ST) is visible on the bottom left of the image. In (b), the cement has been scaled and is no longer attached to the implant and has moved and is only visible on the upper right between the shield and the implant. In both images, the endoscope shield is on the right.

Conclusion

Dental hygiene continues to make advancements toward treating periodontal disease. While the endoscope is not without challenges, it brings many advantages and improvements in the process of scaling and root planing. Hygienists could benefit in many ways by utilizing this technology in a practice setting.

The Use of the Dental Endoscope and Videoscope for Diagnosis and Treatment of Peri-Implant Diseases

5

Thomas G. Wilson Jr.

Overview

Inflammation is frequently found around failed or failing implants. Some feel that these are infections engendered by some of the same bacteria associated with periodontal diseases [1]. Others have suggested that this inflammation is caused at least in part by a foreign body reaction [2]. An inflammatory response limited to the soft tissues surrounding implants is referred to as peri-implant mucositis. If the inflammation results in progressive bone loss, the condition is currently termed "peri-implantitis." These two inflammatory responses are categorized under the super heading of peri-implant disease.

Chapter objectives

This chapter outlines treatments available for peri-implant diseases using minimally invasive procedures. The use of the dental endoscope in diagnosis and the endoscope and videoscope in the treatment of peri-implant disease will be emphasized. Clinical and scientific information currently available indicates that if the inflammation associated with peri-implant mucositis is diagnosed and treated at an early stage, loss of bone may not occur. It should also be understood that our

Minimally Invasive Periodontal Therapy: Clinical Techniques and Visualization Technology, First Edition.
Edited by Stephen K. Harrel and Thomas G. Wilson Jr.
© 2015 John Wiley & Sons, Inc. Published 2015 by John Wiley & Sons, Inc.
Companion Website: www.wiley.com/go/harrel/minimallyinvasive

understanding of these inflammatory processes is at an early stage. It should also be stated that appropriate treatment for periodontal diseases may not be totally applicable to the inflammatory responses seen around dental implants. However, current information suggests that appropriate treatment of peri-implant disease may slow down or in some cases halt further bone loss, although reintegration of the lost bone has not yet been demonstrated in humans [3]. At present, most peri-implantitis is treated in its early stages using flap surgery and in its advanced form by implant removal. However, in some of these cases, the disease can be halted or delayed in the early stages by the use of the dental endoscope alone. The videoscope is suggested for more advanced lesions.

Diagnosis and technique

The diagnosis and treatment of peri-implant diseases begins with gathering appropriate clinical and radiographic information. The current data gathering mimics that used for periodontal diseases. This means that probing depths around implants need to be measured and recorded. Signs of inflammatory changes (bleeding upon probing, suppuration, color changes associated with inflammation, etc.) should be noted and recorded. Periodic right-angle radiographs are also appropriate. Because of the relatively high incidence of peri-implant disease, it is imperative that implants be followed on a regular maintenance schedule. This will allow for the comparison of clinical and radiographic findings over time and enhance the clinicians' ability to determine when treatment beyond routine maintenance therapy should be performed.

Treatment is currently based on the diagnosis and characterization of the inflammatory lesion. Patients who present with clinical signs of inflammation but whose probing depths have not increased and have no radiographic signs of increased bone loss are diagnosed as having peri-implant mucositis. Patients so diagnosed should have their oral hygiene reinforced, the peri-implant space (sulcus) and the implant/restorative surfaces debrided using curettes or ultrasonic devices. Attempts should be made to remove surrounding "granulation" tissue. They are usually placed on chlorhexidine rinse twice a day for 30 days. Some clinicians will elect to place the patient on 7–10 days of broad-spectrum antibiotics at this time; but in the absence of suppuration, this does not appear to be routinely indicated. Evaluation and possible treatment of any occlusal disharmonies on the implant prosthesis is also strongly suggested. The patient should be reevaluated after 30 days. If at that time continued signs of inflammation are detected, further treatment is indicated. In these cases, the use of the dental endoscope will enhance the evaluation and treatment of the subgingival environment and help elucidate the source of peri-implant inflammation.

Individuals who present with increased probing depths or radiographic signs of progressive bone loss are given a diagnosis of peri-implantitis. Aggressive treatment of the underlying cause of these clinical findings is indicated when this diagnosis is made. The endoscope is valuable in both the diagnosis and treatment

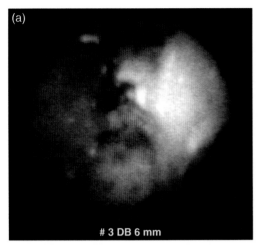
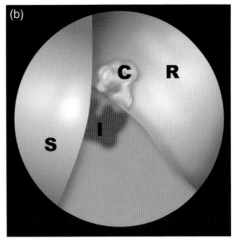

Figure 5.1 An endoscope view (a) and drawing of the field (b). Cement (C) shows up as a highly reflective white areas. Biofilm is usually blue-gray.

of early peri-implantitis and should be employed as soon as feasible on these individuals. However in cases with significant bone loss, the videoscope provides better visibility for removal of "granulation tissue" and foreign bodies.

Endoscopic or videoscopic examination of patients with peri-implant diseases often reveals foreign material attached to the implant surface or to the prosthetic superstructure. The most common finding is a blue-gray film (Figure 5.1) attached to or surrounding the surface of the implant or its superstructure. This material is easily displaced by the tip of the endoscope explorer. It is assumed that this material is a biofilm similar to bacterial plaque found around teeth. White highly reflective material (Figure 5.1) is often seen attached to the implant or its superstructure. This material is dental cement. Subgingival calculus similar to that seen around teeth has never been observed by the author.

After inspection of the implant and the attached superstructure, the endoscopic explorer is rotated 180° and the peri-implant soft tissue (sulcular tissue) is evaluated. Foreign material is often seen in these tissues. This material shows up as very small white dots apparently embedded in the soft tissues. This material represents flecks of cement. Evaluation of human biopsies of soft tissues around implants suffering from peri-implantitis has routinely found deposits of cement and titanium surrounded by inflammatory cells [2].

The use of an endoscope greatly improves the clinicians' ability to debride the area. Current clinical experience in the treatment of peri-implant mucositis indicates that when the endoscope is used to treat the peri-implant inflammation; in a vast majority of cases, this results in a long-term elimination of the clinical manifestations of inflammation.

Individuals with a diagnosis of peri-implantitis present greater challenges. By definition, these individuals have lost bone that is assumed to have been originally attached to the implant surface. Since reattachment of this bone (re-osseointegration) has not been demonstrated in humans, the clinician must decide on the most appropriate treatment based on the circumstances found around each individual implant. Treating early bone loss (<25% of the implant rough surface exposed) with the endoscope can often result in elimination or reduction of the clinical and radiographic signs of inflammation. It should be understood that recession of the soft tissues is likely to occur and this may create esthetic problems. In general, implants with 75% or more of the implant exposed should be removed. The quandary exists for those individuals between these two extremes.

Individuals who have greater than 25% bone loss and less than 75% bone loss can often have the progress of the disease halted (at least in the short term) by removing any implant-borne accretions and surrounding effected soft tissue. The videoscope is suggested for these procedures. This result is apparently because removal of peri-implant soft tissues reduces or eliminates the number of foreign bodies found surrounding the implant. The author's opinion is that most surgical interventions should involve reduction of one- and two-wall bony craters, removal of affected soft tissues, and judicious smoothing of any exposed roughened surface of the implant followed by apical positioning of the flaps [3]. This is because adequate methods for removing biofilm and its products such as lipopolysaccharides from the implant surface have not yet been shown to be predictable. Multiple studies are currently underway on the best way to clean these implant surfaces. Once the best approach (or approaches) has been defined, then the routine use of appropriate hard tissue grafting materials in these cases may be apropos. Until that time, it is suggested that graft materials not be routinely used since their long-term efficacy has not been demonstrated. Again, it should be remembered that surgical procedures for this category of bone loss will result in significant soft tissue recession and exposure of the implant surface.

Description of the mechanics of the procedures to be performed

After a diagnosis of peri-implant disease is made and informed consent obtained, treatment can be initiated.

Treatment of peri-implant mucositis

Only topical anesthetic is usually needed for this procedure. Aided by endoscope visualization, as much of the material adherent to the implant as possible should be removed. While a number of medicaments have been suggested to remove biofilm and its products, at present the author suggests the use of chlorhexidine [4]. It is currently assumed that some bacteria and/or their byproducts will remain on the implant surface. Thus, the need for reinforcing of personal oral hygiene and frequent post-treatment evaluation arises. The most frequently found foreign body on the implant is cement. Once removal of material on the implant surface is accomplished, the endoscope explorer is rotated 180° to view the peri-implant soft tissues. The soft tissue should be curetted with the goal of removing as much "granulation tissue" as possible. The patient is normally placed on chlorhexidine rinse to be used twice a day and an evaluation is scheduled for 30 days later. A broad-spectrum antibiotic such as amoxicillin is occasionally prescribed. At the reevaluation if any signs of inflammation are present, the endoscope should be used again, and this should be repeated until the signs of inflammation are gone. If this does not result in the elimination of the inflammatory process, appropriate evaluation for other local and systemic problems is appropriate.

Treatment of peri-implantitis

In general, the endoscope should be used to diagnose peri-implantitis, and the videoscope should be used to treat it. After flap elevation (see Chapter 7), any accretions on the implant or superstructure are removed. In these cases, aggressive removal of the inflamed peri-implant tissues is appropriate. Again it should be borne in mind that recession of the soft tissues is likely to occur. In these cases, the process of removing implant-borne materials often results in the fragmentation of these accretions and their embedding in the surrounding soft tissues. Since these particles often illicit an inflammatory response, this necessitates careful evaluation of the peri-implant soft tissues before flap closure. Chlorhexidine is usually prescribed and reevaluation is done at 30 days.

It is suggested that clinicians new to minimally invasive procedures restrict their treatment to patients with peri-implant mucositis because of the inherent challenges of removal of foreign bodies both on the implant surface and in the soft tissues seen in cases of peri-implantitis.

The cement problem

The vast majority of the implants receiving single- or multiple-unit fixed partial dentures are seated using dental cement. This approach has been shown to be less technologically challenging and less expensive than using a screw-retained restoration. This has resulted in the overwhelming use of the cemented approach for implant restorations [5]. Along with the ease and facility of this approach comes a very important problem—that of excess cement. This material has often been found on superstructures, implant surfaces, and in the peri-implant tissues and has been shown to be associated with peri-implant disease [6]. Early evidence has shown that it is virtually impossible at cementation to remove all of this luting material from around margins that are placed apical to the gingival marginal tissues [7].

This retention of excess cement may act in a manner similar to calculus seen on natural teeth, in that it concentrates endotoxins that can result in an inflammatory response. Unfortunately, the clinical and radiographic manifestation of this problem often does not occur for years following cementation. This argues strongly for periodic maintenance visits for individuals with cemented dental implant restorations. This is especially true for mixed dentition, individuals who have both natural teeth and implants and whose teeth have periodontitis. These individuals have been shown to have more peri-implant disease than individuals with no remaining natural teeth [8].

Prevention of peri-implant disease secondary to dental cement has four components: (i) proper surgical placement, (ii) proper abutment design, (iii) early removal of excess cement, and (iv) appropriate maintenance for patients.

During surgery, the implant abutment interface should be placed slightly coronal to the gingival tissues to move the cement line to the level of the gingiva that allows for more predictable removal of excess cement. Flattening posterior bony ridges during surgery reduces the soft tissue accumulation seen on the facial/lingual plane of the bony housing that hinders cement removal.

Minimal luting agent should be placed into the fixed partial denture, excess material can be extruded prior to final cementation using a stock abutment analog or a custom analog made from impression material after lining the inside of the crown with Teflon tape. The use of retraction cord or rubber dam material to allow access for excess cement removal is often appropriate. Immediate attempts should be made to evaluate the area around the newly cemented crown for any excess luting material.

Example cases

Case 1

This 34-year-old post-orthodontic patient wanted an implant in the space previously occupied by his mandibular left deciduous molar. This molar had been removed several years before and not replaced. Clinical and radiographic examination revealed absence of this tooth as well as a high mental foramen position in relation to the existing alveolar ridge, thus necessitating the placement of a short implant. An osseointegrated implant was placed uneventfully into the site (Figure 5.2a). This patient was monitored once a year for evidence of peri-implant disease. A clinical and radiographic examination performed 5 years after placement reveals no clinical or radiographic signs of peri-implant disease (Figure 5.2b). Five months later, the patient reported to the office with a chief complaint of swelling around the implant (Figure 5.2c). Probing depths had increased from 3 to 7 mm, and there was radiographic evidence of bone loss on the distal of the implant compared with a radiographic exposed 5 months earlier.

An endoscopic examination was performed using local anesthesia. A small flap was raised and excess cement was seen on the distal of the implant and was removed using ultrasonic devices aided by endoscopic visualization. The area has

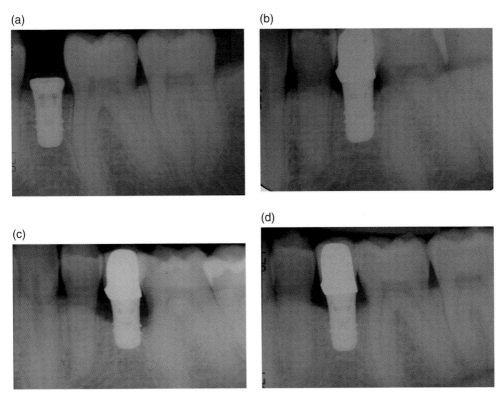

Figure 5.2 (a) This radiograph was exposed immediately after placement of the implant in the mandibular left deciduous molar site. (b) A single-unit cemented fixed partial denture was placed after the implant integrated. (c) The patient reported with a chief complaint of swelling on the distal of the implant. There was a 7-mm probing depth in the area. (d) The area seen radiographically 5½ years after cementation.

remained stable 5 years after an intervention, the distal probing depth is now 4 mm, and there are no clinical signs of peri-implant mucositis, but the bone loss seen radiographically and clinically has not returned to its previous level (Figure 5.2d).

Case 2

This patient presented with a failing fixed partial denture from the mandibular left second molar through the mandibular left second bicuspid. Clinical and radiographic examination revealed an extensive carious lesion on the molar (Figure 5.3a). The molar was removed and two implants placed. The implant in the second molar position was placed as an immediate, and the fixture in the first molar was placed into mature bone (Figure 5.3b). The mesial surface of the second molar implant placed immediately was covered by natural bone, and the exposed distal surface was covered with a hard tissue graft. The implant in the position of the first molar was completely surrounded by mature bone. The

(a)

(b)

(c)

(d)

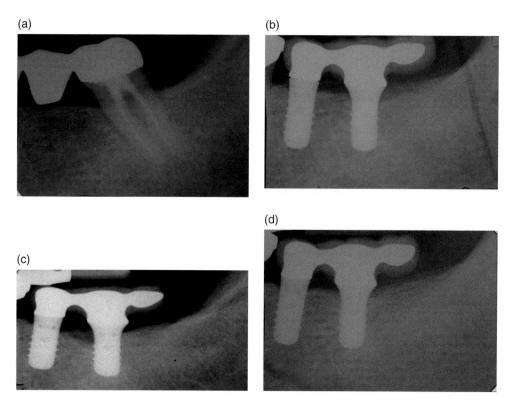

Figure 5.3   (a) This mandibular second molar abutment for a three-unit fixed partial denture had extensive caries and was slated to be removed. (b) The molar was extracted and an implant placed immediately. A second implant was placed into the first molar site. (c) The patient was seen every year to evaluate the implants. Approximately 4 years after implant placemen, the patient presented with radiographic signs of bone loss and clinical signs of inflammation and the mesial of the second molar implant. Relevant history included recent re-cementation of his fixed partial denture. Endoscopy revealed a large deposit of excess cement associated with the lesion. The cement was removed with the help of the endoscope. (d) Following removal of the excess cement, the area showed clinical and radiographic signs of repair.

patient was seen for yearly follow-ups. Four years after placement, the patient presented with suppuration and radiographic bone loss on the mesial of the implant replacing the second molar (Figure 5.3c). The bone loss had occurred on the surface originally encased by mature bone. Relevant clinical history included that the prosthetic superstructure had loosened within the last few months and was re-cemented by his general dentist.

Endoscopic evaluation of the area found a large amount of excess cement on the mesial of the second molar implant that was removed. As a result, the probing depths that had been 7 mm reduced to 3, and the radiographic evidence of bone loss disappeared. This result has been stable for 5 years (Figure 5.3d).

Case 3

This patient is a 55-year-old man. He presented with a failed endodontic treatment on the maxillary left central incisor (Figure 5.4a). Because of the large root form of the tooth and the minimal amount of apical bone available for implant stabilization (Figure 5.4b). Delayed implant placement was chosen as the preferable approach. The tooth was removed and guided bone regeneration (socket enhancement) was performed. Approximately 6 months later, an osseo-integrated dental implant was placed. Following integration, a single-unit fixed partial denture was seated using dental cement. A 6-month post-cementation clinical examination revealed no apparent problems (Figure 5.4c). Two months later, the patient presented with an abscess on the facial of the implant (Figure 5.4d). The abscess had fenestrated the gingival tissue approximately 2 mm apical to the free

(a)   (b)

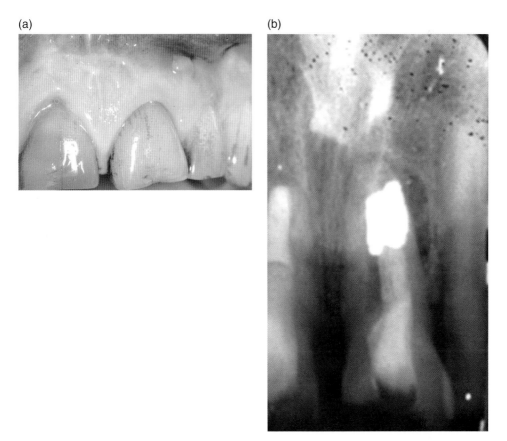

Figure 5.4   (a) This patient's maxillary left central incisor had a failed endodontic lesion. Because of the lack of bony support for a potential implant, the tooth was removed and the socket treated with hard and soft tissue grafting. Six months later, an implant was placed. (b) A preoperative radiograph of the incisor seen in (a).

(c) (d)

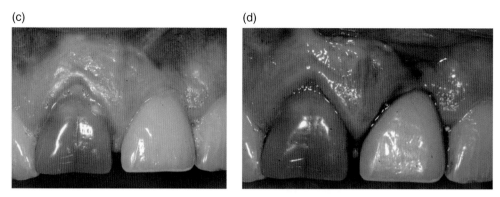

Figure 5.4 (*Continued*) (c) Two months later, the patient presented with an abscess on the facial of the implant. (d) The clinical presentation 8 months after the crown was cemented.

gingival margin. Endoscopy was performed and a small piece (~1/3 mm × 1/3 mm) of cement was visualized and removed. While the signs of peri-implant disease were eliminated, the opening in the soft tissues remains and the peri-implant tissues have been stable for 3 years after treatment (available on the book companion website).

Conclusions

Peri-implant disease is seen in a significant number of implant patients. These inflammatory responses are is in some ways similar to periodontal diseases. Therefore, diagnosis and maintenance procedures are very similar for these problems. It appears that intervention at the mucositis stage and appropriate removal of noxious materials along with adequate personal oral hygiene will often result in elimination of clinical signs of inflammation and prevention of subsequent bone loss in most cases. Peri-implantitis, the progressive loss of bone around the implant, presents a greater challenge for the clinician. Many cases of peri-implant disease are related to excess cement. The early stages of peri-implantitis usually respond well to removal of the noxious materials from the implant and superstructure surfaces and soft tissue debridement. Advanced bone loss around these fixtures is usually best treated by the removal of the implant. At present, individuals with greater than 25% and less than 75% bone loss around their implants present the biggest challenge. Current approaches do not allow us to routinely arrest the progression of bone loss. However, the dental endoscope and videoscope have proved to be invaluable tools in diagnosing and treating these diseases, but it should be understood that the current level of our understanding of these problems and their treatment needs to be expanded.

References

1. Heitz-Mayfield, L.J., Salvi, G.E., Mombelli, A., Faddy, M. & Lang, N.P. (2012) Anti-infective surgical therapy of peri-implantitis. A 12-month prospective clinical study. *Clinical Oral Implants Research*, **23 (2)**, 205–210.
2. Wilson, T.G. Jr., Valderrama, P., Burbano, M., Blansett, J., Levine, R., Kessler, H. & Rodrigues, D.C. 2014. Foreign bodies associated with peri-implantitis human biopsies. *Journal of Periodontology* (in press).
3. Valderrama, P. & Wilson, T.G. Jr. (2013) Detoxification of implant surfaces affected by peri-implant disease: an overview of surgical methods. *International Journal of Dentistry*. Epub August 4, 2013.
4. Valderrama, P., Blansett, J.A., Gonzalez, M.G., Cantu, M.G., & Wilson, T.G. Jr. (2014) Detoxification of implant surfaces affected by peri-implant disease: an overview of non-surgical methods. *The Open Dentistry Journal*, **8**, 77–84.
5. Jung, R.E., Pjetursson, B.E., Glauser, R., Zembic, A., Zwahlen, M. & Lang, N.P. (2008) A systematic review of the 5-year survival and complication rates of implant-supported single crowns. *Clinical Oral Implants Research*, **19 (2)**, 119–130.
6. Wilson, T.G. Jr. (2009) The positive relationship between excess cement and peri-implant disease: A prospective clinical endoscopic study. *Journal of Periodontology*, **80 (9)**, 1388–1392.
7. Linkevicius, T., Vindasiute, E., Puisys, A. & Peciuliene, V. (2011) The influence of margin location on the amount of undetected cement excess after delivery of cement-retained implant restorations. *Clinical Oral implants Research*, **22 (12)**, 1379–1384.
8. Sgolastra, F., Petrucci, A., Severino, M., Gatto, R. & Monaco, A. (2013) Periodontitis, implant loss and peri-implantitis. A meta-analysis. *Clinical Oral Implants Research*. doi: 10.1111/clr.12319 [Epub ahead of print].

6 Development of Minimally Invasive Periodontal Surgical Techniques

Stephen K. Harrel

All treatments for periodontal diseases are centered, at least in part, on the thorough debridement of the root surfaces. Without the removal of plaque, biofilm, and calculus from the root surfaces, most authorities agree that periodontal treatment whether aimed at ameliorating the disease process or the regeneration of lost periodontal tissue is doomed to failure. Bearing this goal in mind, all periodontal surgical approaches are aimed at allowing the surgeon improved access and visualization to debride root surfaces and the periodontal lesion.

Most authorities credit Widman and Neumann with the first descriptions of periodontal surgery [1,2]. The surgery described involved large incisions to expose the bone beyond the apex of the teeth, allowing for the debridement of root surfaces and osseous defects. Often, it was recommended that the interproximal bone be left exposed to allow for the formation of new interproximal tissue. This surgical technique was aimed at pocket elimination. Everett credits Kirkland with describing the first periodontal surgical procedures that were aimed at regeneration and reattachment to the root surface [3]. Most traditional periodontal surgical procedures are modifications of these early techniques.

Schluger was the first to described periodontal osseous surgery [4]. Osseous surgery had many similarities to the original procedure described by Widman but altered the treatment of the bone by reshaping the alveolar bone to include the removal of existing osseous defects. Ramfjord described what he termed the modified Widman procedure [5]. This procedure also had many of the elements

Minimally Invasive Periodontal Therapy: Clinical Techniques and Visualization Technology, First Edition.
Edited by Stephen K. Harrel and Thomas G. Wilson Jr.
© 2015 John Wiley & Sons, Inc. Published 2015 by John Wiley & Sons, Inc.
Companion Website: www.wiley.com/go/harrel/minimallyinvasive

of the original Widman procedure but utilized a much more conservative flap design and did not include the complete surgical removal of osseous defects.

Despite many strongly held opinions at the time these surgeries were current, traditional periodontal flap surgery techniques whether aimed at pocket elimination or amelioration had many similarities. Most used large incisions that allowed for the reflection of the tissue from around many teeth. Typically, the flap reflection included all or most of the teeth in a quadrant to gain access to the underlying defects. In addition, a frequent end point was some amount of apical positioning of the gingival tissue.

The advent of surgery aimed at the regeneration of periodontal supporting tissue began a change in periodontal surgical techniques that resulted in a move toward minimally invasive periodontal surgery. Most credit Hyatt and Schallhorn with the introduction of bone grafting techniques for periodontal regeneration [6]. The original surgical techniques for periodontal regeneration were very similar to those that were in use at the time for pocket elimination procedures. As regenerative surgical techniques became established, the size of the surgical access gradually became smaller and more localized. Often vertical releasing incisions were used to allow for a more localized access to an area of bone loss. However, relatively large localized flaps continue to remain the norm for most regenerative periodontal procedures.

One of the first descriptions of a small flap procedure was termed "mini-flap" [7]. A mini-flap, by definition, was the reflection of the papilla to allow for better access for root planing. The gingival papilla was reflected and root planing was performed with the assistance of fiber optic illumination. The papillae were repositioned with pressure from saline-soaked gauze only. No sutures were used. The mini-flap procedure was viewed as an enhancement for root planing and as a method to fully remove sulcus epithelium. The authors did not describe regeneration of periodontal supporting tissue as a major goal of the treatment method. The 24-month post-operative data indicated approximately 1.8 mm in improved calculated attachment level as well as 0.8 mm of gingival recession. This represented a moderate improvement over the results obtained from traditional closed root planing without the use of the mini-flaps.

The first description of a periodontal surgical procedure that was described as minimally invasive was in 1995 [8]. The paper described a surgical instrument that allowed for the debridement of periodontal defects through very small access incisions. This minimally invasive technique was further developed over the next several years as a surgical technique for periodontal regeneration using bone grafts and other regenerative materials. The periodontal surgical technique was described as Minimally Invasive Surgery for periodontal regeneration and is referred to as MIS [9]. This technique and later modifications are fully described and referenced in Chapter 7. In 2007, another minimally invasive surgical technique for periodontal regeneration was described. This technique was based on the papilla preservation technique and was described as the Minimally Invasive Surgical Technique and is referred to as MIST [10]. This technique and later modifications are fully described and referenced in Chapter 8. A minimally invasive approach for the treatment of soft tissue defects utilizing a tunnel procedure for the placement of soft tissue grafts is described and referenced in Chapter 9.

The current minimally invasive surgical techniques that utilize small incisions for the treatment and regeneration of the destruction caused by periodontal disease can be seen as the result of an evolution that has occurred over the entire history of surgical periodontal treatment. Today, we are able to treat and regenerate periodontal destruction through surgical openings that would have been unimaginable as little as 30 years ago. The data presented in Chapters 7, 8, and 9 indicate that not only are we able to obtain excellent regeneration that is very stable over a long time period, but this regeneration is possible with much reduced patient morbidity, and unaesthetic results are minimized or eliminated. Improvements in technology for visualization are a major force in the ability to perform minimally invasive periodontal regeneration. As technology continues to improve, it is very likely that surgical access openings will continue to become smaller and regenerative results are likely to improve. Some of the potential future changes in minimally invasive periodontal techniques are discussed in Chapter 10.

References

1. Widman, L. (1918) The operative treatment of pyorrhea alveolaris. A new surgical method. Sv. Tandl. Tidsk., December.
2. Neumann, R. (1920) *Die Alveolarpyorrhoe und ihre Behandlung*, 3rd edn. Hermann Meusser, Berlin, Germany.
3. Everett, F.G., Waerhaug, J. & Widman, A. (1971) Leonard Widman: Surgical treatment of pyorrhea alveolaris. *Journal of Periodontology*, **42**, 571.
4. Schluger, S. (1949) Osseous resection: A basic principal in periodontal surgery. *Oral Surgery, Oral Medicine, Oral Pathology*, **2**, 361.
5. Ramfjord, S. & Nissle, R. (1974) The modified Widman flap. *Journal of Periodontology*, **45 (8)**, 601–607.
6. Schallhorn, R., Hiatt, W. & Boyce, W. (1970) Iliac transplants in periodontal therapy. *Journal of Periodontology*, **41 (10)**, 566–580.
7. Reinhardt, R., Johnson, G. & Tussing, G. (1985) Root planing with interdental papilla reflection and fiber optic illumination. *Journal of Periodontology*, **56**, 721–726.
8. Harrel, S.K. & Rees, T.D. (1995) Granulation tissue removal in routine and minimally invasive surgical procedures. *Compendium of Continuing Education in Dentistry*, **16**, 960–967.
9. Harrel, S.K. (1998) A minimally invasive surgical approach for bone grafting. *The International Journal of Periodontics & Restorative Dentistry*, **18**, 161–169.
10. Cortellini, P. & Tonetti, M.S. (2007) Minimally invasive surgical technique and enamel matrix derivative in intra-bony defects. I: *Clinical outcomes and morbidity*. *Journal of Clinical Periodontology*, **34**, 1082–1088.

7 The MIS and V-MIS Surgical Procedure

Stephen K. Harrel

Introduction

Minimally invasive surgery (MIS) is based on the concept of using small incisions to perform surgical procedures that have previously been performed through larger surgical access openings. The term "minimally invasive surgery" was first applied to periodontal surgical procedures in 1995 [1]. The procedure was described as minimally invasive surgery or MIS. Several variations and techniques for performing MIS have been described. These include the original MIS approach that used surgical telescopes for visualization, a variation of this approach using the glass fiber endoscope for visualization, and the most recently described technique of Videoscope-Assisted MIS (V-MIS). Each of these techniques is considered to be an MIS technique with each change in visualization technology, thereby allowing for smaller incisions and greater magnification.

Following the initial description of MIS, the technique was further explored in several case series published over the next five years [2–5]. These papers reported excellent clinical results over an extended time period. The largest of these case series had 194 surgical sites that were followed for 9–54 months. All patients had closed scaling and root planing performed under local anesthetic at least 6 week before the surgical procedure. At the time of surgery, the pockets to be surgically treated ranged from 5 to 16 mm. The mean improvement in pocket

Minimally Invasive Periodontal Therapy: Clinical Techniques and Visualization Technology, First Edition.
Edited by Stephen K. Harrel and Thomas G. Wilson Jr.
© 2015 John Wiley & Sons, Inc. Published 2015 by John Wiley & Sons, Inc.
Companion Website: www.wiley.com/go/harrel/minimallyinvasive

probing depth was 4.58 mm, and the mean improvement in clinical attachment level (CAL) was 4.87 mm. A detailed description of the technique for performing MIS was published in 1999 [3].

Further research on MIS has been published more recently. A prospective study of the use of MIS with enamel matrix derivative (EMD) was published with 1-year data in 2005, and the 6-year data on the same cases published in 2010 [6,7]. These studies showed that there was a significant amount of improvement in pocket probing depth and CAL when MIS was performed. A total of 160 sites were treated with EMD using an MIS approach. The presurgical pocket probing depths following closed subgingival scaling and root planing were 5 mm or greater with a range of 5 mm–12 mm. At 1 year and at 6 years, the mean pocket probing depths were 3.09 mm and 3.06 mm, respectively. The mean improvement in CAL at 1 and 6 years post surgery was 3.33 mm and 3.36 mm, respectively. All pocket probing depths were less than 4 mm at all reevaluations. One of the most clinically significant findings in this study was the lack of clinically detectable recession at both measurement intervals. Recession is a major concern associated with all types of periodontal surgery. The lack of recession following MIS is an important finding because it indicates that the risk of unaesthetic gingival contours, food impaction, and thermal sensitivity is minimal following MIS regenerative surgery.

Recently, a videoscope has been designed for use with MIS [8,9]. This videoscope was described in Chapter 2. The use of the videoscope has allowed for smaller surgical access openings when performing MIS, and the procedure is described as Videoscope-Assisted Minimally Invasive Surgery V-MIS. A large university based study of V-MIS indicates that there is a further improvement over MIS when V-MIS is used. The mean presurgical pocket probing depths following closed subgingival scaling and root planing were 5.23 mm with a mean CAL of 5.86 mm and 0.82 mm of recession. At 6 months following V-MIS, the mean pocket probing depth was 2.28 mm while all pocket probing depths were less than 3 mm. There was an improvement in CAL of 3.00 mm. There was also a small, but statistically significant, improvement in soft tissue height of 0.29 mm [10]. This study further emphasizes that the MIS and specifically the V-MIS surgical technique yield good improvement in pocket probing depths and CAL while not causing clinical and esthetic complications associated with recession. The surgical technique described in this chapter will be based on the V-MIS approach to minimally invasive surgery.

Surgical principles

There are certain principles that guide all MIS procedures. The first is to preserve as much blood supply to the periodontal tissues as possible. Preserving the blood supply means that split thickness dissection is used for all flap reflection and a periosteal elevator is never used. This is a critical aspect of MIS. A major source of blood supply for the periodontal tissues is the periosteum. The reflection of the periosteum with a perosteal elevator significantly disturbs the blood supply to the gingival tissue and underlying bone. Care should be taken to leave the periosteum intact. The bone should only be exposed within the defect itself. A second principle of MIS is to cause minimum traumatic damage to the periodontal tissue. In most traditional regenerative periodontal surgery, it is routine to make large flaps and widely reflect the soft tissue from the bone. With MIS, care is taken to use as small an incision as possible, use split thickness dissection to reflect the soft tissue only to the edge of the osseous defect, and to put as little pressure on the tissue as possible. When successful, at closure the tissue should have the appearance of the surrounding un-incised tissue and to not have a bruised or cyanotic appearance. A third principle of MIS is to replace the soft tissue at or above the presurgical height with no tension on the tissue. Suturing is kept as simple as possible, and sutures are only placed at the base of the flap. The thin coronal portion of the papilla is never penetrated with a needle as it is felt this negatively impacts the blood supply to this thin vulnerable tissue. Instead of suturing the papilla, the tissue is approximated and positioned coronally by finger pressure on wet gauze. The use of the videoscope allows for smaller incisions and flaps that do not have to be reflected to the extent necessary with other means of visualization which aids closure of the tissue.

Steps in V-MIS or MIS

The surgical technique for MIS using either telescopes or a glass fiber endoscope and V-MIS using a videoscope is similar in many ways. The following description will detail the use of a videoscope for V-MIS. The same steps can be followed for MIS using surgical telescopes or a surgical microscope. With V-MIS, smaller access incisions and less flap reflection can be used than with traditional MIS surgical approaches. Major variations in technique necessitated by different visualization technology will be noted in the steps as they are described.

Case selection

V-MIS/MIS is usually indicated for isolated defects. Standard nonsurgical treatment (oral hygiene instruction, closed subgingival scaling and root planing, and occlusal adjustment where appropriate) should be performed prior to making a decision on the type of surgical approach that may be necessary. Often following nonsurgical treatment, a patient who initially presented with generalized periodontal inflammation will instead present with most pocket probing depths at an acceptable level for the maintenance of periodontal health. However, there will frequently be isolated, usually interproximal, defects that are 5 mm or greater in pocket probing depth. (Figure 7.1) The radiographs of these areas should be carefully evaluated and a decision made whether bone loss is present and if so are regenerative procedures indicated. If the defects are localized and are adjacent to periodontally healthy tissue, these defects are the ideal sites for using V-MIS.

		1			2			3			4			5			6		
Pocket					3	2	3	7	3	3	3	2	3	3	3	3	3	2	3
Attachment					3	3	3	7	4	3	3	3	3	3	4	3	3	2	3
GM					0	1	0	0	1	0	0	1	0	0	1	0	0	0	0
Furcation																			
Bleeding																			
Mobility																			
MG INV																			
Plaque																			

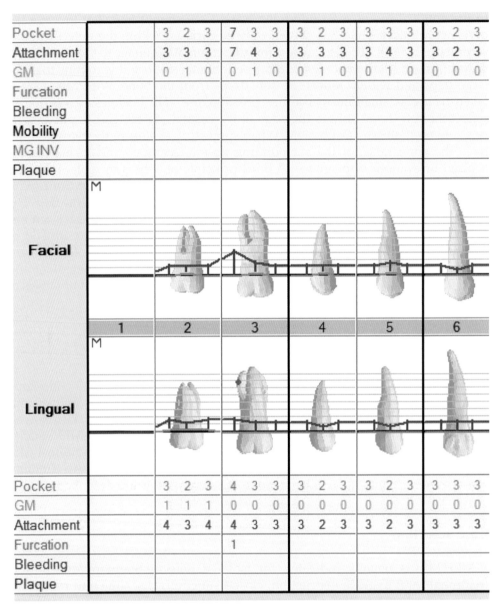

		1			2			3			4			5			6		
Pocket					3	2	3	4	3	3	3	2	3	3	2	3	3	3	3
GM					1	1	1	0	0	0	0	0	0	0	0	0	0	0	0
Attachment					4	3	4	4	3	3	3	2	3	3	2	3	3	3	3
Furcation								1											
Bleeding																			
Plaque																			

Figure 7.1 Charting of a quadrant where V-MIS is indicated. Pocket probing depth chart post initial preparation indicating an isolated defect between the first and second molar. This isolated defect is ideally indicated for a V-MIS/MIS approach.

In cases where the periodontal destruction is more generalized with many contiguous areas of deeper pocket probing depths, it may not be possible to use a minimally invasive approach as it has been described in the literature. (Figure 7.2) However, many of the principles described for use with minimally invasive surgery such as smaller flaps and minimizing trauma to the tissue can still be used for

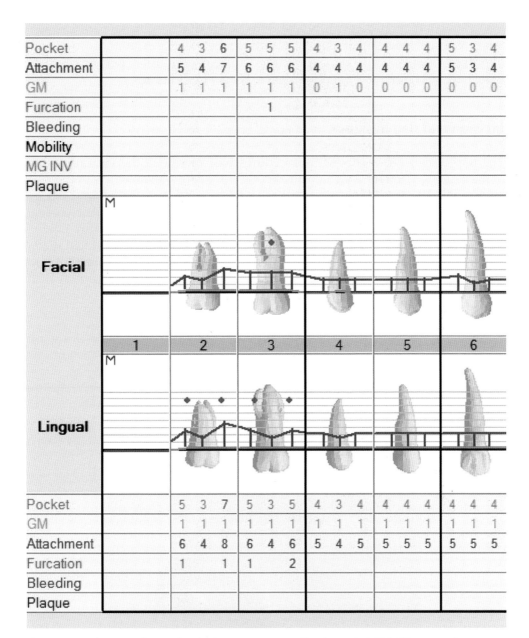

		Tooth 2			Tooth 3			Tooth 4			Tooth 5			Tooth 6		
Pocket		4	3	6	5	5	5	4	3	4	4	4	4	5	3	4
Attachment		5	4	7	6	6	6	4	4	4	4	4	4	5	3	4
GM		1	1	1	1	1	1	0	1	0	0	0	0	0	0	0
Furcation						1										
Bleeding																
Mobility																
MG INV																
Plaque																

Facial

1   2   3   4   5   6

Lingual

		Tooth 2			Tooth 3			Tooth 4			Tooth 5			Tooth 6		
Pocket		5	3	7	5	3	5	4	3	4	4	4	4	4	4	4
GM		1	1	1	1	1	1	1	1	1	1	1	1	1	1	1
Attachment		6	4	8	6	4	6	5	4	5	5	5	5	5	5	5
Furcation		1		1	1		2									
Bleeding																
Plaque																

Figure 7.2 Charting of a quadrant where more generalized (non-V-MIS/MIS) surgery is indicated. Pocket probing depth chart post initial preparation showing generalized defects that indicate the need for a more generalized surgical approach than V-MIS/MIS. Small incision surgery and the use of the videoscope will be of benefit for this case, but more extensive (longer) incisions will be necessary.

the treatment of more generalized periodontal damage despite the necessity for a more extensive reflection of tissue. The videoscope because of its ability to provide improved visualization and magnification can be very useful in performing these more generalized (nonminimally invasive) surgical procedures.

Incision and flap design

The flap design for V-MIS/MIS procedures will vary with the location, extent of the osseous defect, and visualization devices that are available. The presence of an osseous defect can be diagnosed with routine pocket measurements, but the extent of bone loss should be verified by bone sounding after the patient has been anesthetized. Where possible, only a single lingual or palatal flap is used. Lingual access and visualization is much easier when a videoscope is available. Lingual access approaches are difficult to use when surgical telescopes or a surgical microscope are used. These instruments give a straight view into the surgical field, which means a mirror must be used with a lingual flap approach. By contrast, the

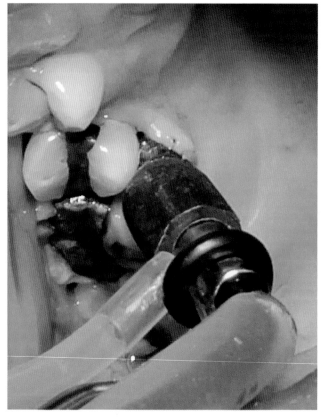

Figure 7.3   The videoscope is placed through a single MIS access flap on the palate allowing for full visualization of the interproximal defect.

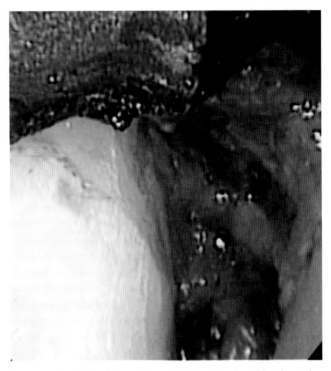

Figure 7.4   The interproximal defect from Figure 7.3 as visualized by the videoscope.

videoscope can be placed directly into the lingual opening, which results in a clear view of the surgical site. (Figures 7.3 and 7.4)

Assuming an interproximal defect that does not extend beyond the line angles of adjacent teeth, the first incision is placed in the intersulcular space from the line angle of each tooth extending into the interproximal area. Care should be taken to stay in the sulcus and not remove a collar of tissue with this incision (Figure 7.5). This requires that the blade be placed against the tooth and pushed to the base of the defect. The blade should not be allowed to incise the tissue in the body of the papilla, and care should be taken to not cross the body of the papilla with these incisions. The second incision should be a horizontal (mesial-distal) incision across the body of the papilla (Figure 7.6). This incision should be placed relatively high on the papilla but not extend into the area of the col. The col should be preserved in place if at all possible. Once the horizontal incision is made, a split-thickness dissection is performed to create the access flap (Figure 7.7). This should be done only with sharp dissection. A periosteal elevator should never be used to elevate this flap.

Various blades can be used for making these incisions. The following suggestions for blades are those used by the author. The initial sulcular incisions are made with a 12b blade (Figure 7.8). This is a standard curved disposable scalpel blade where both edges of the curve are sharpened. This blade has the advantage of some rigidity and the ability to be utilized in a push–pull motion. This has been

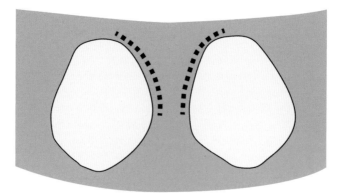

Figure 7.5 An outline drawing of the initial sulcular incisions. These initial incisions are made in the sulcus of the teeth adjoining the periodontal defect. The incisions are kept strictly within the sulcus by placing the blade against the adjacent root surface. No collar of tissue is removed with this incision, and care is taken to not join the two incisions.

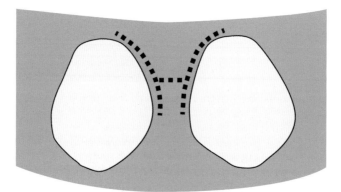

Figure 7.6 An outline drawing of the incision jointing the two sulcular incisions across the papilla. The two initial incisions are connected on the surface (buccal or lingual) where the access flap will be elevated. This connecting incision is made apical to the col tissue. The col tissue and the papilla on the nonsurgical side remain intact and are not elevated.

found to be very useful for the sulcular incisions. This blade may also be used to make the horizontal incision across the body of the papilla. The sharp dissection of the papilla is performed with a modified Orban knife. A standard Orban knife is reduced in size by approximately one third of its width (Figure 7.9). The rigidity of the Orban knife is very helpful for reflecting the flap because it allows for a split thickness dissection as well as the ability to "pull" on the flap as the incision is made. Other blades that may be helpful are the so-called microsurgical blades (Figure 7.10). The size of these blades allows good access to small spaces, but the blade's lack of rigidity is often a significant impediment to their use. These blades also tend to have a "spring" that causes the blade to move suddenly when the blade "catches" on bone or calculus. This sudden movement of the very sharp blade may damage the tissue.

(b)

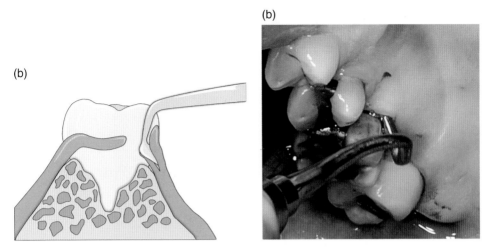

Figure 7.7   (a) Outline drawing of using a modified Orban knife to reflect the access flap. The access flap is reflected with sharp dissection only leaving the periosteum in place on the bone. A periosteal elevator should not be used. Because of its rigidity, a small Orban knife is ideal for this step. (b) Clinical use of a modified Orban knife for the sharp dissection.

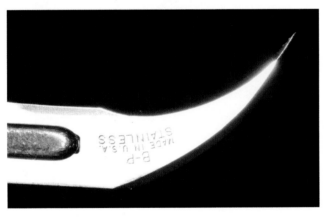

Figure 7.8   Because of its push–pull cutting capabilities and its relative rigidity, a disposable 12b blade is ideal for making the initial sulcular incisions and the incision across the papilla.

If a videoscope is not available or if the osseous defect is extensive, it may be advisable to create a buccal flap in addition to the lingual minimal access flap. When telescopes or a surgical microscope is used, consideration can also be given to using only a buccal approach. However, it should be borne in mind that reflecting a buccal flap has a greater potential for visible gingival recession with possible negative esthetic consequences.

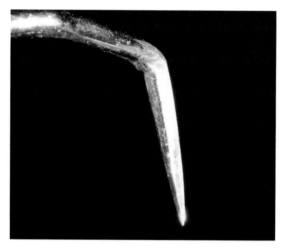

Figure 7.9   A standard Orban knife modified by reducing its width by approximately one third is ideal for making the split thickness incision that is used to elevate the access flap. The rigidity of this blade allows for the cutting of the tissue and also displacing flap for access.

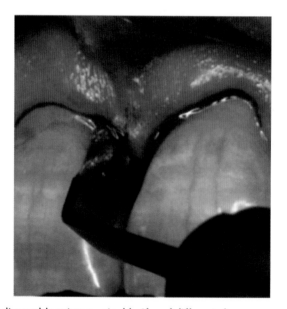

Figure 7.10   Many disposable microsurgical knifes of different shapes are available, which can be used for all the incisions used in V-MIS/MIS. Because the shafts of these knifes are very flexible, they may not be ideal for some steps in making V-MIS/MIS incisions.

Debridement

A through debridement of the periodontal defect and adjacent tooth is necessary for optimal chances of regeneration. Debridement of the defect consists of two parts. The first is the removal of granulation tissue. The second is the removal of calculus, biofilm, and surface roughness from the root surface.

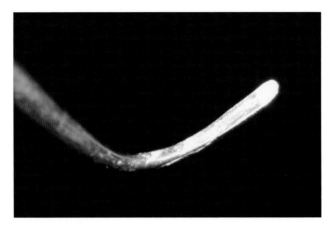

Figure 7.11   The blade of a Younger-Goode 7/8 curette is ideal for the gross removal of granulation tissue from periodontal defect through the small MIS access opening. This curette can be utilized in a manner similar to an operative "spoon" instrument used to remove caries.

The debridement of granulation tissue from the defect is performed using standard periodontal curettes. Larger curettes such as a Prichard curette are too large for use in most V-MIS procedures. Care should be taken to keep from placing pressure on or folding the soft tissue flap while debriding the defect. This means that most traditional periodontal retractors are not suitable for use in MIS. If a videoscope is available, the rotating carbon fiber tissue retractor will adequately retract the V-MIS flap without causing damage to the soft tissue. If a videoscope is not available, great care should be taken to not apply excessive pressure when retracting the flap for visualization as this will damage the tissue and lead to postsurgical recession. The instrument most used for granulation tissue removal with V-MIS/MIS is a Younger-Goode 7–8 (Figure 7.11). This is a relatively small instrument with a narrow shaft that can be used in a motion similar to a "spoon" used for the removal of decay. This motion is far less likely to place excess pressure on the minimal flap than will the standard root planing like motion used in traditional periodontal surgery. Other small curettes can also be used, but the prevention of damage to the soft tissue flap should be a goal throughout debridement.

Classically, all granulation tissue is removed during periodontal surgery. With high magnification, this can become an extremely difficult job. This is especially true when the videoscope with 40+ magnification is used. The author's goal is to remove as much granulation tissue as possible from next to the tooth and from the floor of the defect. The granulation tissue on the soft tissue walls (Figure 7.12) is removed to a point that allows for visualization of the root surface, but the definitive removal of "all granulation tissue" is not pursued.

The debridement of the root surface is usually started with an ultrasonic scaler. The Diamond Safety Tip (Vista Dental, Milwaukee, WI) is the preferred ultrasonic tip for this (Figure 7.13). This tip brings the aggressiveness of a diamond ultrasonic tip; but because the abrasive action of the diamond is limited, it can safely be used in small defects without risk of damaging the root surface. Following the

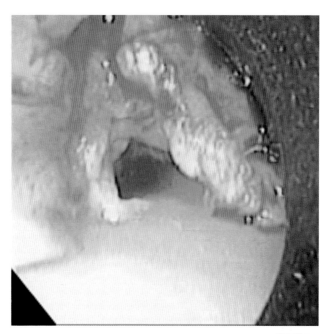

Figure 7.12 Photo of a surgical defect with granulation tissue removed illustrating the intact col tissue and the unreflected buccal papilla. Granulation tissue is removed from the osseous defect and a "tunnel" is made under the unreflected papilla. Tags of granulation tissue remaining on the unreflected tissue and on the underside of the access flap are removed only to the extent necessary to visualize the defect.

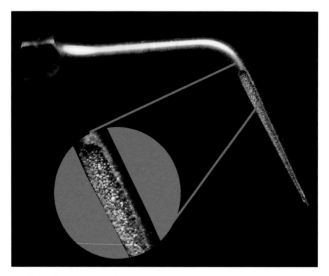

Figure 7.13 Initial debridement of the root surface is performed with an ultrasonic scaler. The Diamond Safety Tip (Vista Dental) is preferred for this step. It allows for the rapid removal of calculus and roughness with the diamond abrasive, but it does not cause any damage of the root surface.

use of an ultrasonic scaler, hand curettes, typically Graceys, are used for the mechanical removal of the remaining calculus. Care must be taken to clean and dry the surgical area before visualizing the root surface with the videoscope for remaining calculus. This drying is best accomplished by packing a strip of dry gauze into the site and withdrawing the gauze just before placing the videoscope in place.

With V-MIS, when the mechanically debrided root surface is observed with the videoscope, there will often be "micro" islands of calculus remaining, which are not observable with telescopes or the surgical microscope (Figure 7.14). These micro islands of calculus are usually not detectable with a periodontal probe. These small areas of calculus can be very difficult to remove by mechanical means. The use of biomodification with either ethylenediaminetetracetic acid (EDTA) or citric acid will usually remove all of the remaining islands of calculus (Figure 7.15). The author feels this final removal of microcalculus is extremely important to the long-term results reported for MIS and V-MIS.

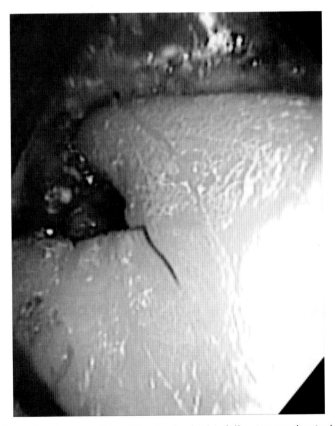

Figure 7.14 Photo showing remaining islands of calculus following mechanical root debridement. After mechanical debridement of the root surface with ultrasonic and hand curettes, the videoscope will often reveal "micro islands" of calculus that remain on the root surface.

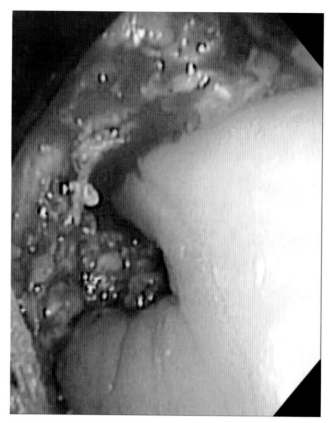

Figure 7.15   The root surface shown in Figure 7.14 after the use of ethylenediaminetetraacetic acid (EDTA). Note that the micro islands of calculus seen in Figure 7.14 are no longer present.

Regenerative materials

Most of the MIS and V-MIS cases reported in the periodontal literature have used either enamel matrix derivative (EMD) alone or mixed with freeze-dried demineratized cortical human bone allograft (DFDBA). However, the author has performed V-MIS/MIS using only EMD, only DFDBA, and with no regenerative material. The use of each of these approaches has led to similar excellent clinical results. Cortellini has reported that if the blood supply to the surgical site is well maintained, no regenerative materials are necessary with small incision surgery (MIST) [11,12]. The author agrees with this observation in many instances. This is probably most true when the lesion is relatively small and narrow and, therefore, supports the soft tissue. If the lesion is somewhat larger, the use of DFDBA, with or without EMD, will help support the flap and prevent it from sinking into the underlying defect. This seems to be beneficial in preventing recession and postsurgical esthetic problems. The use of EMD appears to speed the soft tissue healing of the flaps and has been associated with long-term stability of periodontal regeneration. Based on these clinical considerations, the use

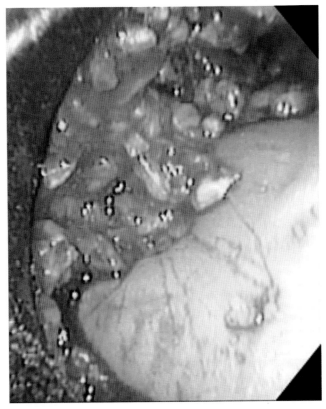

Figure 7.16   Photo showing freeze-dried particulate bone graft material mixed with enamel matrix derivative (EMD) placed in the periodontal osseous defect. The use of a growth stimulator such as EMD in association with a material to support the flap such as freeze-dried demineralized human bone appears to be ideal for use in V-MIS/MIS regeneration.

of EMD both on the root surface and mixed with DFDBA when flap support is needed seems to be an ideal approach (Figure 7.16).

The small opening used in V-MIS precludes the use of a membrane for cellular exclusion. One of the principles of guided tissue regeneration is to extend the occlusive membrane several millimeters beyond the edge of the osseous defect. This would negate much of the advantages gained from the use of small incisions. This extension also would necessitate the exposure of a considerable amount of bone with the subsequent loss of blood supply from the area denuded of periosteum. In the early descriptions of MIS, a technique was discussed in which a Vicryl mesh was placed over a bone graft in the osseous defect. This mesh material was dead soft with relatively large holes in the material. The Vicryl mesh was not placed for cellular exclusion but for stabilization of the bone graft and subsequent blood clot. The use of a Vicryl membrane has been discontinued with no apparent changes in clinical results. The author no longer recommends this step for MIS or V-MIS.

Suturing

A single suture is used for the typical closure of a V-MIS site. In most cases, the material used is either a 4-0 plain collagen or chromic suture. However, the exact suture material does not appear critical, but it should be strong enough to allow the tissue to be pulled firmly together and not be so small that it cuts through the tissue when tension is applied. A vertical mattress suture is placed at the base of papilla (Figure 7.17). The suture is placed in this position so that tension can be placed on the suture without fear of damaging the papillary tissue in a manner that might cause postoperative recession. The suture at the base of the papilla will allow the body of the papilla to be pulled firmly together without damaging the thin and narrow tissue at the apex of the papilla. Suturing coronal to the base of the papilla, even with very small suture and fine needles, is avoided in order to not damage this vulnerable tissue. It is felt that this suturing technique that avoids trauma to the papillary tissue is one of the major reasons that no mean recession is reported following V-MIS/MIS.

The papilla tissues coronal to the suture are approximated by placing saline-soaked gauze on the tissue and applying finger pressure (Figure 7.18). Where possible, the interproximal soft tissue is placed at or above the presurgical level.

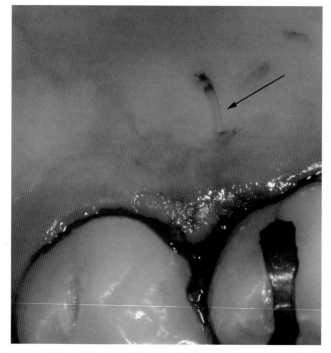

Figure 7.17 The access flap is closed with a simple vertical mattress suture placed at the base of the papilla. Sutures are not placed through the tip of the papilla in order to not damage the blood supply to this thin tissue.

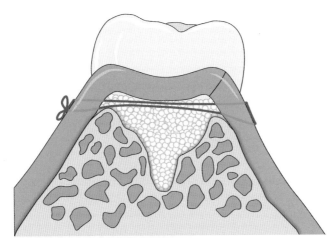

Figure 7.18   After the base of the papilla has been closed with a vertical mattress suture, the tips of the papilla are approximated at or above the presurgical height with finger pressure only.

This will help minimize the possibility of postsurgical recession, which is one of the significant advantages of the V-MIS/MIS procedure.

Postoperative instructions

Patients generally require only over-the-counter pain medication such as Ibuprofen or Acetaminophen following surgery. They are advised to avoid mechanical oral hygiene in the surgical area for 7–10 days and to use chlorhexidine mouth rinses twice a day. A 5–7 day course of broad spectrum antibiotic can be prescribed for postsurgical use if the surgeon feels this is necessary. A moderately soft diet is recommended for 1 week following surgery.

Most patients report little pain or other morbidity following MIS. Often, the patients will say they forget that surgery has been done and brush or chew routinely in the surgical area despite being advised not to do so. While this can certainly lead to complications, it is an indication that the patient has little discomfort following MIS.

Summary

Minimally invasive surgery using the very small incisions of V-MIS or using the somewhat larger incisions of MIS has a proven track record of producing shallow pocket probing depths, improved attachment levels, clinically undetectable recession, and long-term stability of the improved results following surgery. In addition to these favorable clinical results, patient satisfaction with these procedures has been high. This is reflected in a lack of discomfort immediately following the surgical procedure, no food packing, or thermal sensitivity following initial surgical healing, and minimum to no negative esthetic changes following surgery. The use of V-MIS/MIS where indicated for regeneration of damage from periodontal destruction is highly clinically predictable and is viewed very favorably by patients.

The video link to *Journal of Clinical Periodontology* (Wiley) "pubcast" is available on the book companion website.

Case Study 1

A 53-year-old Caucasian female presented with chronic moderate-to-severe generalized periodontal disease. Initial therapy consisted of oral hygiene instruction, nonsurgical root planing with local anesthetic, and reevaluation at 6 weeks post root planing. At the time of reevaluation, most pocket probing depths had returned to an acceptable level of 4 m or less. However, multiple isolated interproximal sites with pocket probing depths of 5–8 mm remained. These sites were treated with V-MIS.

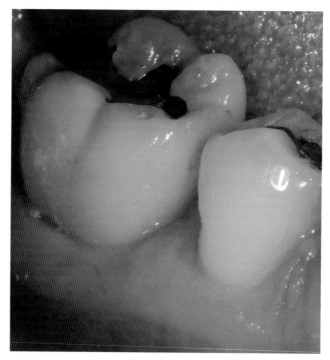

Figure CS1 7.1 Presurgical buccal view of the surgical area. A pocket of 8+ mm remained interproximally between the first molar and second bicuspid, following initial therapy consisting of root planing with local anesthetic.

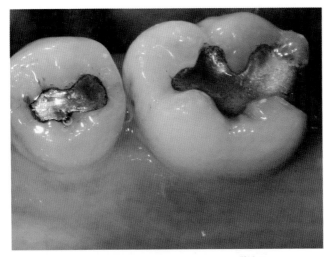

Figure CS1 7.2   Presurgical lingual view of the surgical area pictured in Figure CS1 7.1.

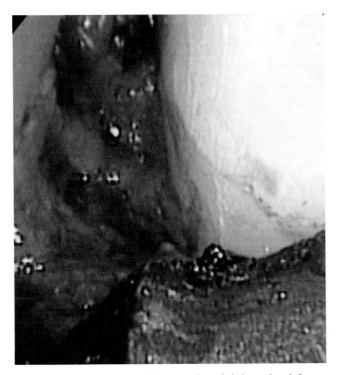

Figure CS1 7.3   Initial videoscope view of the periodontal defect. The defect was accessed using only a lingual MIS access incision.

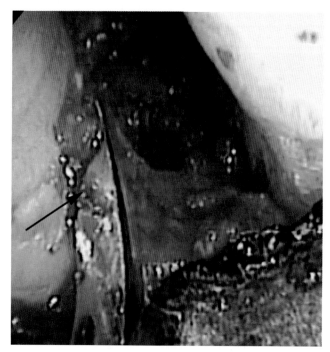

Figure CS1 7.4 Videoscope view of the periodontal defect showing the use of a Younger-Goode curette (arrow) to remove granulation tissue. Note the apparent vascular channel present in the bony wall of the periodontal defect.

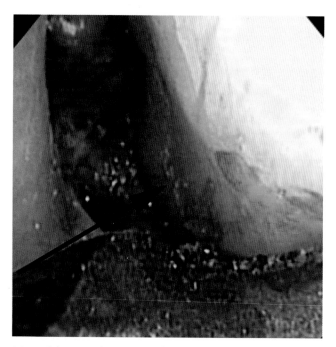

Figure CS1 7.5 Most of the granulation tissue has been removed, and the root surfaces have been mechanically debrided of all calculus visible with surgical loupes, and no roughness could be detected with a periodontal probe. When the lesion is visualized with the videoscope "micro" islands of calculus are visible (arrow).

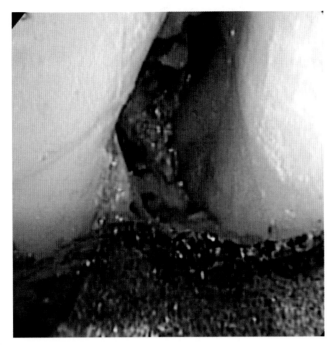

Figure CS1 7.6   The root surface has been treated with EDTA to biomodify the roots surface. The micro islands of calculus are no longer visible.

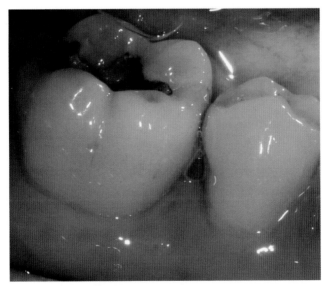

Figure CS1 7.7   A buccal view of the surgical area at 6 month post surgery.

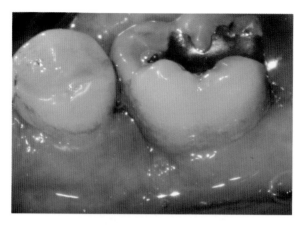

Figure CS1 7.8 A lingual view of the surgical area at 6 months post surgery. No measurable recession is noted.

Case Study 2

The patient is a 54-year-old man who presented with generalized moderate and locally severe periodontitis. He responded well to nonsurgical periodontal therapy consisting of root planing with local anesthetic. Most pocket probing depths returned to an acceptable level of 4 mm or less. Several sites continued to have deeper pocket probing depth, gingival inflammation, and bleeding on probing. These areas were treated nonsurgically with the use of a periodontal endoscope

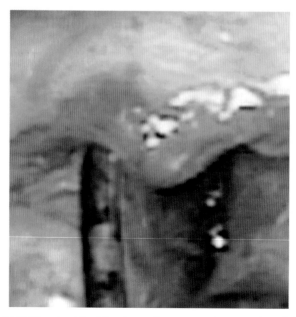

Figure CS2 7.1 A V-MIS palatal incision is used to access the periodontal defect.

(Perioview). All areas responded well to this therapy with the exception of a single site between a maxillary first molar and second bicuspid. This site had a residual 7-mm pocket probing depth and continued bleeding on probing. The site was treated with V-MIS, bone grafting, and enamel matrix derivative.

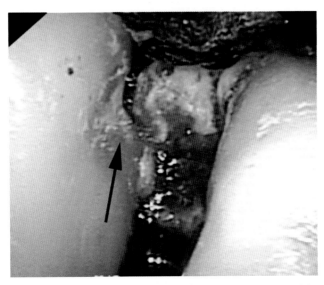

Figure CS2 7.2   Videoscope view of the periodontal lesion with a portion of the granulation tissue removed. Note the calculus filled "depression" on the interproximal aspect of the distal tooth. All other root surfaces had been rendered calculus free by the two nonsurgical procedures.

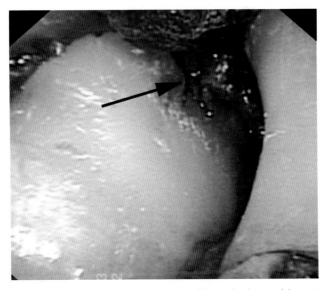

Figure CS2 7.3   Further granulation tissue and most of the calculus visible in Figure CS2 7.2 has been removed. Dark calculus extending to the level of the bone is now revealed.

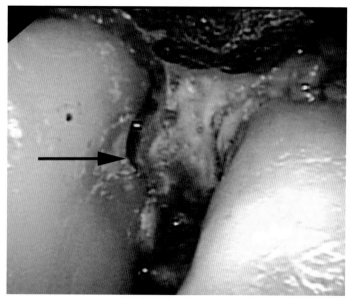

Figure CS2 7.4 All granulation tissue has been removed and the bony floor of the periodontal defect is visible. The depression on the root with remaining calculus is fully visible.

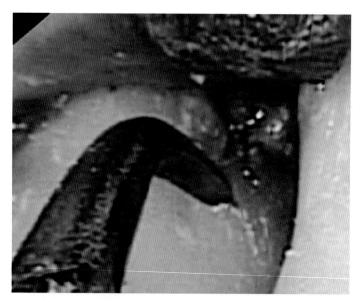

Figure CS2 7.5 Mechanical removal of the remaining calculus being performed with a Gracey curette. Following mechanical removal of calculus, multiple micro islands of calculus were observed with the videoscope. EDTA was used to remove the remaining calculus and to biomodify the root surface.

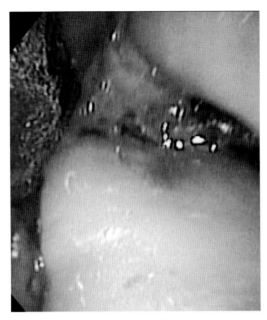

Figure CS2 7.6 The root surface following the use of EDTA. At this point, EMD and DFDBA were placed in the defect and the access flap was closed.

At six months post operative, the site has a pocket probing depth of 3 mm, no bleeding on probing, and no clinically detectable postsurgical gingival recession.

V-MIS Gallery

Diagnosis and root abnormalities identified with the videoscope

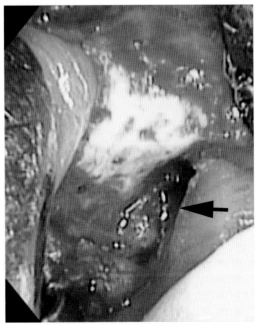

Figure G7.1 Root resorbtion detected in a maxillary molar bifurcation defect.

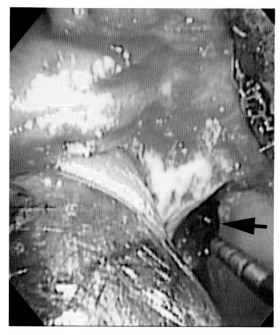

Figure G7.2 The root resorbtion noted in Figure G7.1, following clean out. At patient's request, the lesion was filled with a glass ionomer and the lesion was bone grafted. At 9 months post surgery, the area had healed well.

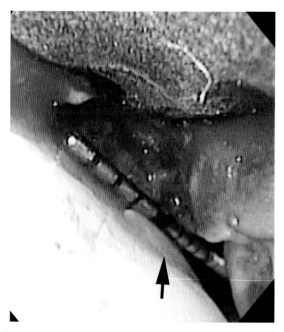

Figure G7.3 Enamel pearl located on the root surface approximately 2 mm apical to the CEJ. This root abnormality was smooth and undetectable to a periodontal probe prior to surgical access and the removal of the small amount of planed calculus that surrounded the enamel pearl.

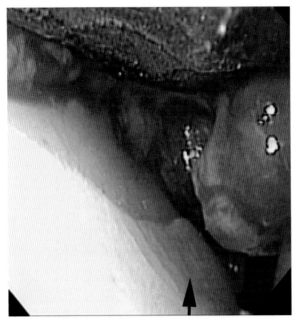

Figure G7.4   The root surface pictured in Figure G7.3, following the removal of the enamel pearl and root biomodification with EDTA. The pearl was removed with diamond-coated ultrasonic scalers and smoothed with a rotary carbide finishing burs.

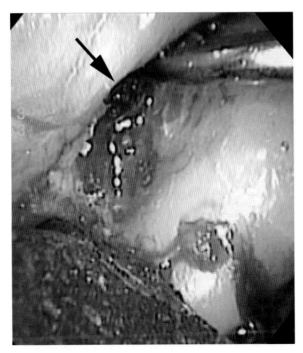

Figure G7.5   Root decay is noted apical to the CEJ. The instrument in the illustration is inserted into the area of decay.

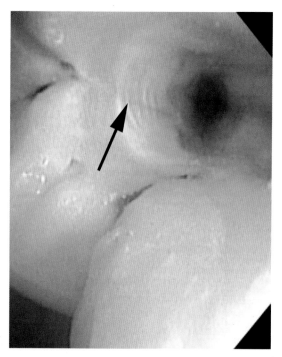

Figure G7.6 The pulp chamber has been opened and a fracture of the pulp chamber wall is verified with the videoscope. Based on this finding the tooth was extracted and the site prepared for an implant.

Cement on implants

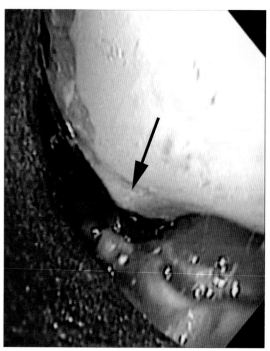

Figure G7.7 Excess cement at the base of an implant supported crown is identified by the use of the videoscope.

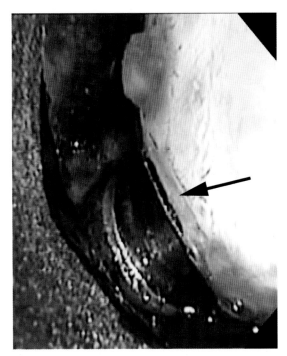

Figure G7.8 The excess cement has been removed with the exception of a thin line at the crown margin (arrow). The surgical site has been prepared to attempt regeneration of bone and reattachment to the implant. The soft tissue will be positioned apical to the crown margin.

Calculus on root surfaces

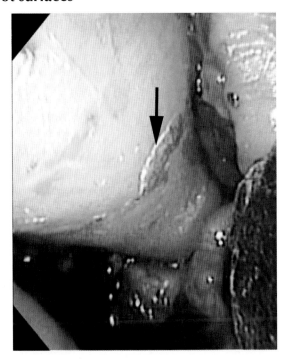

Figure G7.9 An isolated area of calculus is visualized on the mid-lingual surface of the root. The remainder of the root had been planed free of calculus during closed root planing and the calculus shown was very smooth and undetectable with a probe when the root was palpated prior to surgery.

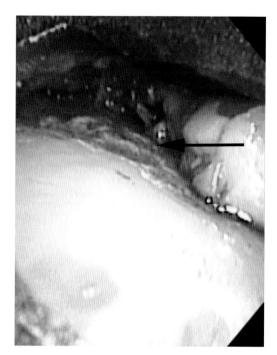

Figure G7.10 Area of deep calculus visualized at the base of a large periodontal defect. All surrounding root surface had been planed smooth during nonsurgical root planing, but the deepest area of the defect appeared untouched.

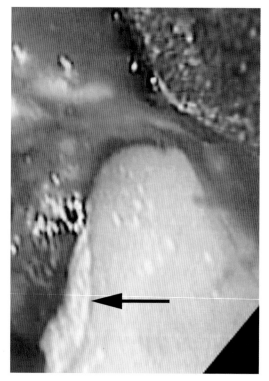

Figure G7.11 A large area of smooth "burnished' calculus is visualized on the distal root surface. The calculus had been planed smooth during many episodes of root planing over several years.

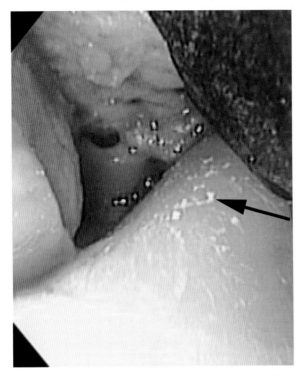

Figure G7.12 The calculus seen in Figure G7.11 has been removed with ultrasonic instruments and hand scalers. Note that many micro islands of calculus remain.

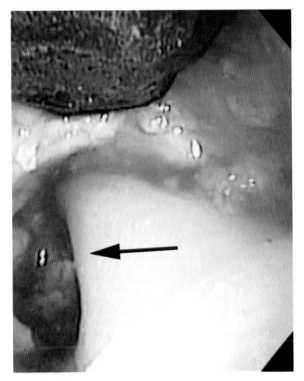

Figure G7.13 The root surface shown in Figure G7.12, following biomodification by the use of EDTA. Note that the micro islands of calculus are no longer present.

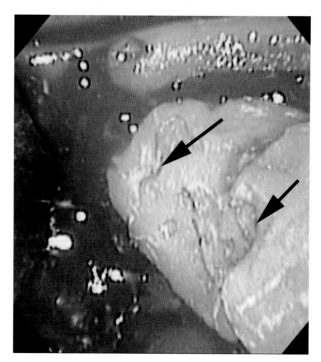

Figure G7.14 A root surface exposed during V-MIS showing calculus present in many depressions on the root surface. The cause of these root irregularities is unknown.

"Lines" on root surfaces

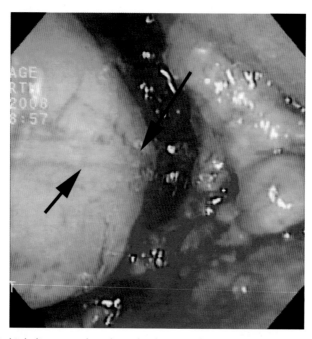

Figure G7.15 Multiple lines noted on the palatal root surface on a maxillary central incisor. When first noted, these lines were filled with dark calculus, and it was assumed the tooth was fractured. However, as the root was scaled it was determined that there were multiple linear depressions in the root surface. It is unknown if these depressions are natural or part of the disease process.

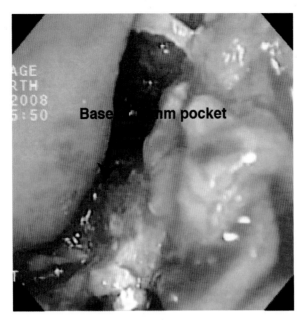

Figure G7.16 The root surface shown in Figure G7.15 after root planing with diamond ultrasonic scalers and hand curettes, followed by biomodification with citric acid. At 2 years post operative, the pocket probing depth had been reduced from 10 mm preoperatively to 3 mm post operative. Post-operative recession was approximately 1 mm.

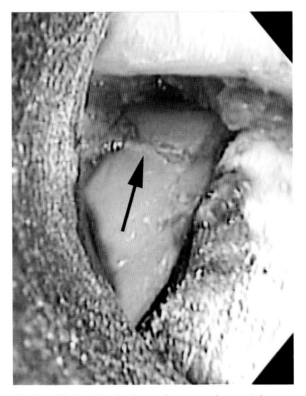

Figure G7.17 A single line filled with calculus is shown on the mesial root surface of a maxillary bicuspid. When the line was removed with a scaler, no fracture of the root could be detected.

Treatment of a maxillary molar bifurcation defect

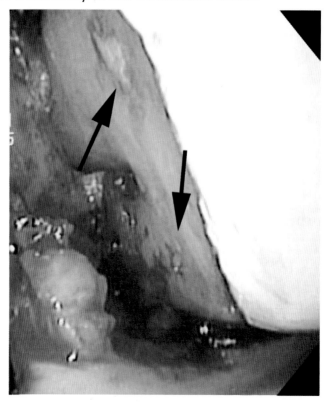

Figure G7.18 An interproximal periodontal lesion on the mesial of a maxillary molar with a class II bifurcation defect. Generalized sheet calculus is noted on the root surface and in the bifurcation.

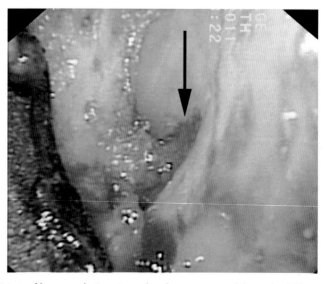

Figure G7.19 Most of he granulation tissue has been removed from the bifurcation defect, and the root surface has had most of the calculus removed.

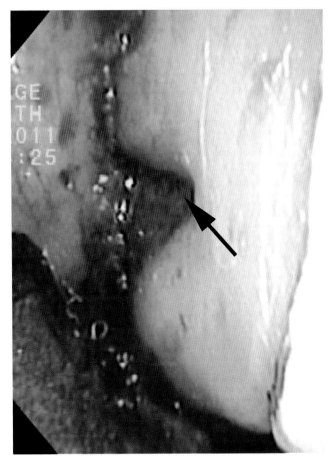

Figure G7.20   Removal of granulation tissue from the bifurcation and mechanical debridement of the root surface has been completed. The use of EDTA has removed the remaining micro islands of calculus. EMD and DFDBA were placed in the defect, including the bifurcation. At 3 years post operatively, the bifurcation defect cannot be probed.

References

1. Harrel, S.K. & Rees T.D. (1995) Granulation tissue removal in routine and minimally invasive surgical procedures. *Compendium of Continuing Education in Dentistry*, **16**, 960–967.
2. Harrel, S.K. (1998) A minimally invasive surgical approach for bone grafting. *The International Journal of Periodontics & Restorative Dentistry*, **18**, 161–169.
3. Harrel, S.K. (1999) A minimally invasive surgical approach for periodontal regeneration: Surgical technique and observations. *Journal of Periodontology*, **70**, 1547–1557.
4. Harrel, S.K., Nunn, M. & Belling, C.M. (1999) Long-term results of a minimally invasive surgical approach for bone grafting. *Journal of Periodontology*, **70**, 1558–1563.
5. Harrel, S.K. & Wright, J.M. (2000) Treatment of periodontal destruction associated with a cemental tear using minimally invasive surgery. *Journal of Periodontology*, **71**, 1761–1766.

6. Harrel, S.K., Wilson, T.G. Jr. & Nunn, M.E. (2005) Prospective assessment of the use of enamel matrix derivative with minimally invasive surgery. *Journal of Periodontology*, **76**, 380–384.
7. Harrel, S.K., Wilson, T.G. Jr. & Nunn, M.E. (2010) Prospective assessment of the use of enamel matrix proteins with minimally invasive surgery: Six year results. *Journal of Periodontology*, **81**, 435–444.
8. Harrel, S.K., Wilson, T.G. Jr. & Rivera-Hidalgo, F. (2013) A videoscope for use in minimally invasive periodontal surgery. *Journal of Clinical Periodontology*, **40**, 868–874.
9. Harrel, S.K., Hidalgo-Rivera, F. & Abraham, C. (2012) Tissue resistance to soft tissue emphysema during M 8. *Journal of Contemporary Dental Practice*, **13** (6), 886–891.
10. Harrel, S.K., Abraham, C.M., Rivera-Hidalgo, F., Shulman, J. & Nunn, M. (2014) Videoscope-assisted minimally invasive periodontal surgery (V-MIS). *Journal of Clinical Periodontology, DOI:***10**.1111.
11. Cortellini, P. & Tonetti, M.S. (2007) Minimally invasive surgical technique and enamel matrix derivative in intra-bony defects. I: *Clinical outcomes and morbidity. Journal of Clinical Periodontology*, **34**, 1082–1088.
12. Cortellini, P. & Tonetti, M.S. (2009) Improved wound stability with a modified minimally invasive surgical technique in the regenerative treatment of isolated interdental intrabony defects. *Journal of Clinical Periodontology*, **36**, 157–163.

8 Minimally Invasive Surgical Technique and Modified-MIST in Periodontal Regeneration

Pierpaolo Sandro Cortellini

Introduction

Periodontal regenerative technologies are applied to improve short- and long-term clinical outcomes of periodontally compromised teeth, presenting with deep pockets and reduced periodontal support. The persistence of deep pockets following active periodontal therapy has been associated with an increased probability of tooth loss in patients attending supportive periodontal care programs [1]. Teeth with deep pockets associated with deep intrabony defects are considered a clinical challenge: periodontal regeneration has been shown to be effective in the treatment of one-, two-, and three-wall intrabony defects or combinations thereof, from very deep to very shallow, from very wide to very narrow [2–5]. Therefore, the application of regenerative procedures, including minimally invasive procedures, is suited in deep and shallow intrabony defects.

Regeneration is a healing outcome that can occur when the systemic and local conditions are favorable. The systemic conditions include the control of periodontitis, a low total bacterial load in the mouth and cessation of smoking habits: high percentages of bleeding on probing and high bacterial loads as well as cigarette smoking have been associated with reduced clinical outcomes [6–12]. The local conditions include the presence of space for the formation of the blood clot at the interface between the flap and the root surface [12–17], the stability of the

Minimally Invasive Periodontal Therapy: Clinical Techniques and Visualization Technology, First Edition.
Edited by Stephen K. Harrel and Thomas G. Wilson Jr.
© 2015 John Wiley & Sons, Inc. Published 2015 by John Wiley & Sons, Inc.
Companion Website: www.wiley.com/go/harrel/minimallyinvasive

blood clot to maintain a continuity with the root surface avoiding formation of a long junctional epithelium [13,18–20], and the soft tissue protection to avoid bacterial contamination [10,21–23].

Development of periodontal regenerative medicine in the past 25 years has followed two distinctive, though totally interlaced paths. The interest of researchers has thus far focused on regenerative materials and products on the one side and on novel surgical approaches on the other side.

In the area of materials and products, three different regenerative concepts have been explored: (i) barrier membranes, (ii) grafts, and (iii) wound healing modifiers, plus many combinations of the aforementioned concepts [5].

In general, the development of surgical procedures was aimed at complete preservation of the soft tissues to achieve and maintain primary closure on top of the applied regenerative material/substance during the critical early stages of healing. Specifically, flap designs attempted to achieve passive primary closure of the flap combined with optimal wound stability.

In the 1990s, the modified papilla preservation technique (MPPT)[15] and the simplified papilla preservation flap (SPPF)[24] have been tested and proposed. These clinical innovations in flap design and handling have radically changed surgery and have allowed a drastic limitation of interdental wound failure to less than 30% of the treated cases. Further enhancements of clinical outcomes were achieved when an operative microscope was adopted [25,26]. Authors reported an increased capacity to manipulate the soft tissues that resulted in an improved potential for primary closure of the wound to an excellent 92% obtained with microsurgery. Other authors reported improved outcomes using operative microscopes in different areas of periodontal surgery, from flap surgery to mucogingival surgery [27–32].

In the past decade, a growing interest for more friendly, patient-oriented surgery have urged clinical investigators to focus their interest in the development of less invasive approaches [33–35]. Following this path, Cortellini and Tonetti proposed a minimally invasive surgical technique (MIST) on isolated [36] and multiple [37]intrabony defects, and a Modified MIST (M-MIST)[38] on isolated intrabony defects.

Clinical studies and outcomes

Cohort studies and randomized controlled clinical trials reporting outcomes on the application of minimally invasive surgical approaches are reported in Tables 8.1 and 8.2.

Table 8.1 refers to MIST studies in which the interdental papillary tissues have been elevated to uncover the interdental space completely. This approach is supported by three cohort studies [36,37,39] and two controlled studies [40,41].

Table 8.2 reports studies in which the access to the defect was gained through the elevation of a small buccal flap, without elevation of the interdental papilla. This approach is supported by a cohort study [38] and three controlled studies [42–44]. Interestingly, the cited randomized clinical trials performed using

Table 8.1 Minimally invasive surgical technique (MIST): clinical studies.

MIST	Type of study (quality of evidence)	Interventions	No. pax	No. defects	CAL gain	PD reduction	Δ REC
Cortellini and Tonetti [36]	Case cohort (level 2)	MIST + EMD	13	13	4.8 ± 1.9	4.8 ± 1.8	0.1 ± 0.9
Cortellini and Tonetti [39]	Case cohort (level 2)	MIST + EMD	40	40	4.9 ± 1.7	5.2 ± 1.7	0.4 ± 0.7
Cortellini et al. [37]	Case cohort (level 2)	MIST + EMD	20	44	4.4 ± 1.4	4.6 ± 1.3	0.2 ± 0.6
Ribeiro et al. [40]	RCT (Level 1)	MIST	15	15	2.82 ± 1.19*	3.55 ± 0.88*	0.54 ± 0.58*
		MIST + EMD	14	14	3.02 ± 1.94*	3.56 ± 2.07*	0.46 ± 0.87*
Ribeiro et al. [41]	RCT (level 1)	MIST	14	14	2.85 ± 1.19*	3.51 ± 0.90*	0.48 ± 0.51*
		MINST (RPL)	13	13	2.56 ± 1.12*	3.13 ± 0.67*	0.45 ± 0.46*

MINST, minimally invasive non surgical technique (RPL with the aid of a microscope); MIST, minimally invasive surgical technique.
*No statistical difference.

Table 8.2 Modified-minimally invasive surgical technique (M-MIST): clinical studies.

M-MIST/SFA	Type of study	Interventions	No. pax	No. defects	CAL gain	PD reduction	Δ REC
Cortellini and Tonetti [38]	Case cohort	M-MIST + EMD	15	15	4.5 ± 1.4	4.6 ± 1.5	0.07 ± 0.3
Cortellini and Tonetti [42]	RCT	M-MIST	15	15	4.1 ± 1.4*	4.4 ± 1.6*	0.3 ± 0.6*
		M-MIST + EMD	15	15	4.1 ± 1.2*	4.4 ± 1.2*	0.3 ± 0.5*
		M-MIST + EMD + BioOss	15	15	3.7 ± 1.3*	4.0 ± 1.3*	0.3 ± 0.7*
Trombelli et al. [43]	RCT	SFA	12	12	4.4 ± 1.5*	5.3 ± 1.5*	0.8 ± 0.8*
		SFA + HA + GTR	12	12	4.7 ± 2.5*	5.3 ± 2.4*	0.4 ± 1.4*
Mishra et al. [44]	RCT	M-MIST	12	12	2.6 ± 0.8*	3.8 ± 0.9*	0.5 ± 0.5*
		M-MIST + rhPDGF-BB	12	12	3.0 ± 0.9*	4.2 ± 0.6*	0.8 ± 0.6*

M-MIST, modified minimally invasive surgical technique; SFA, single flap approach; rhPDGF-BB, recombinant human platelet derived growth factor.
*No statistical difference.

minimally invasive surgical approaches (with or without papilla elevation) do not report any difference in terms of clinical outcomes between the minimally invasive control flap approach and the test in which a regenerative material/product was introduced under the flap. The reported outcomes raise a series of hypotheses that focus on the intrinsic healing potential of a wound when ideal conditions are provided with the surgical approach. In other words, the outcomes of these studies challenge clinicians with the possibility to obtain substantial clinical improvements without using products or materials applying surgical techniques that do enhance *per se* blood clot and wound stability. In particular, the advanced flap design of the M-MIST greatly enhances the potential to provide space and stability for regeneration by leaving the interdental papillary soft tissues attached to the root surface of the crest-associated tooth and by avoiding any palatal flap elevation. The interdental soft tissues are the stable "roof" of a room where the blood fills in and forms a clot. The hanging papilla prevents the collapse of the soft tissues, thereby maintaining space for regeneration. The anatomic bone deficiencies are potentially supplemented by the peculiar flap design that provides additional "soft tissue walls" to the missing bony walls improving stability: walls of the "room" are the residual bony walls, the root surface, and the buccal/lingual soft tissues. The minimal flap extension and elevation also minimizes the damages to the vascular system favoring the healing process of the tiny soft tissues.

Clinical indications and diagnostic procedures

Delivering periodontal surgery in general and regenerative treatment in particular requires knowledge, skills, experience, and a well-defined step-by-step approach.

The first step of periodontal therapy is always cause-related therapy, aimed at obtaining patient compliance, reduction of oral bacterial loads, and control of gingival infection.

At completion of nonsurgical cause-related therapy, patients have to be carefully reevaluated. A full periodontal evaluation should be performed to check for (Flow chart 8.1) the following aspects:

1. The compliance of the patient in terms of plaque control: a very low load of bacterial plaque is a major goal of cause-related therapy and key to periodontal regeneration. Optimal regenerative outcomes have been reported in patients keeping full-mouth plaque score lower than 15% [5].
2. The control of periodontal infection: low level of bleeding on probing is another major goal of cause-related therapy and is again extremely important for the regenerative approach. Optimal regenerative outcomes have been reported in patients having full-mouth bleeding score lower than 15% [5].
3. The presence of residual pockets or furcations: after successful nonsurgical phase, most of baseline increased pocket probing depths should have been resolved or greatly reduced.

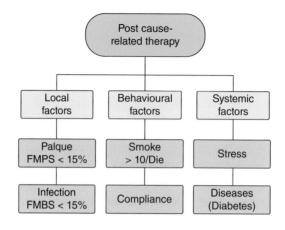

Chart 8.1

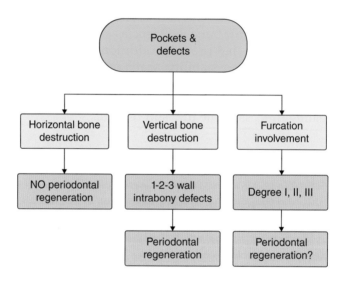

Chart 8.2

4. Additional goals of cause-related therapy are control of behavioral and systemic conditions, such as smoking habits, stress, and systemic diseases (e.g., diabetes).

The presence of residual deep pocket probing depths might indicate the need for periodontal surgery. Surgical treatment of pockets can follow different paths from flap surgery, to resective surgery, to regenerative/reconstructive surgery. Clinical goals of regenerative surgery are to (i) reduce pocket probing depth through attachment gain while limiting the gingival recession and (ii) increase the functional support of the involved teeth. However, periodontal regeneration is not always applicable [5] (Flow chart 8.2). Ample evidence shows that it is highly predictable in the treatment of pockets associated with deep and shallow intrabony defects. Its applicability to furcations is questioned by the scientific community: good outcomes are reported only for the treatment of degree II furcations on lower molars. At present, there is no evidence supporting the application of periodontal regeneration to pockets associated with horizontal bone destruction.

Intrabony defects have been classified according to their morphology in terms of residual bony walls, width of the defect (or radiographic angle), and in terms of their topographic extension around the tooth [45]. Three-wall, two-wall, and one-wall defects have been defined on the basis of the number of residual alveolar bone walls. Frequently, intrabony defects present a complex anatomy consisting of a three-wall component in the most apical portion of the defect, and two- and/or one-wall components in the more superficial portions. Such defects are frequently referred to as combination defects. It is therefore mandatory to clearly diagnose the type of bone defect associated with the pocket. This assessment is based on periodontal probing. The presence of an interproximal intrabony defect is anticipated when there is a difference in the interproximal attachment level between two neighboring teeth. This difference represents the intrabony component of the defect: if the mesial surface of a tooth has an attachment level of 10 mm and the distal surface of the neighboring tooth has an attachment level of 4 mm, the depth of the intrabony component is 6 mm (Figure 8.1a–d). The diagnosis has to be confirmed with a periapical radiograph that provides relevant information about the morphology of both the defect and the root. However, in many instances, the radiograph underestimates the real depth of the defect.

When the presence of an intrabony defect is confirmed, the morphology and extension of the defect and/or the presence of additional defects at neighboring teeth should be carefully inspected. Bone sounding under local anesthetic is highly recommended as a very predictable diagnostic tool to get sound information on the extension of bone destruction.

(a)　　　　　　　　　　　　　　　　　　(b)

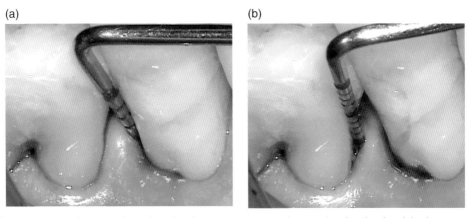

Figure 8.1   (a) The periodontal probe shows a 10 mm pocket on the distal side of the lower right second premolar. (b) A probing depth of 4 mm is detected at the mesial side of the lower right first molar.

(c)   (d)

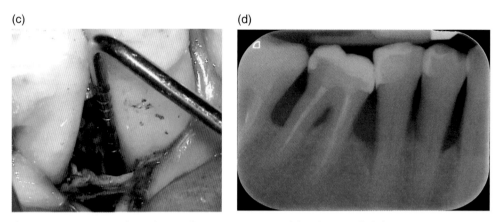

Figure 8.1 (*Continued*) (c) The intrabony component of this three-wall defect is 6 mm. (d) Radiographic image of the intrabony defect.

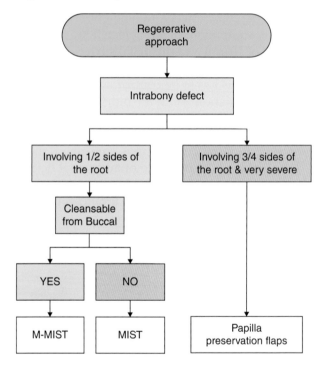

Chart 8.3

    This accurate diagnosis is necessary to select the type of surgical approach and the regenerative materials to be applied to the given clinical condition. In fact, different surgical approaches have been developed through time, which incorporate clear differences in terms of flap design and suturing technique. All the proposed surgical techniques have a common foundation in the attempt to fully preserve the defect-associated interdental papillae and all the buccal and lingual keratinized gingiva by applying intrasulcular incisions. The traditional papilla preservation flaps [15,24] are large and very mobile flaps that allow for ample accessibility and visibility of the defect area, for easy application of biomaterials and barriers, and for the coronal positioning of the buccal flap to cover barriers and biomaterials. The MIST [36], on the contrary, was designed to mobilize just the defect-associated papilla and to reduce flap extension as much as possible. The Modified-MIST [38], based on the elevation of a tiny buccal flap, further enhanced this concept by avoiding the interdental papilla as well as the palatal flap dissection and elevation.

The flow chart 8.3 indicates how to select the flap design according to the defect morphology and extension. Whenever a bone defect involves one or two sides of a root and is cleansable from a small buccal window, an M-MIST can be applied. If such a defect is not cleansable from the buccal window, the interdental papilla is elevated applying a MIST approach. A large papilla preservation flap (MPPT or SPPF), extended to the neighboring teeth and including also a periosteal incision and/or vertical releasing incisions, will be chosen in the presence of a very severe and deep defect, involving three or four sides of the root, requiring ample visibility for instrumentation and the placement of biomaterials and/or barriers.

Minimally invasive surgical technique

The MIST [36,39] is based on the elevation of the defect-associated interdental papilla along with minimally extended buccal and lingual flaps.

The entry incision is performed on the buccal side of the interdental papilla that is dissected with two different approaches according to the width of the interdental space. The width of the interdental space is measured with a periodontal probe as the distance between the two root surfaces; the periodontal probe is positioned horizontally about 2 mm apical to the tip of papilla. In some instances the interdental space is uneven on the buccal and on the lingual/palatal aspect: for example, frequently, the interdental space between the upper cuspid and the bicuspid is narrower on the palatal side than on the buccal one. In these instances, the measurement has to be taken on the palatal side.

In narrow interdental spaces (<2 mm), a buccal diagonal cut is selected, as described in the simplified papilla preservation flap (SPPF)[24]. This incision starts in the interdental sulcus of the defect-associated tooth: the microblade runs toward the contact point, strictly intrasulcular, then crosses diagonally the interdental papilla as close as possible to the papilla tip (the contact point is the limit for the interdental intrasulcular advancement of the blade); the blade cuts through the papilla, hitting the root surface of the crest-associated tooth (Figure 8.2a and b).

Conversely, a buccal horizontal cut is performed in wide interdental spaces (≥2 mm), according to the modified papilla preservation technique (MPPT) [7,15]. The incision is performed through the buccal interdental tissues about midway between the tip and the base of the papilla, keeping the microblade 90° with respect to the gingival surface (Figure 8.3a and b).

(a)   (b)

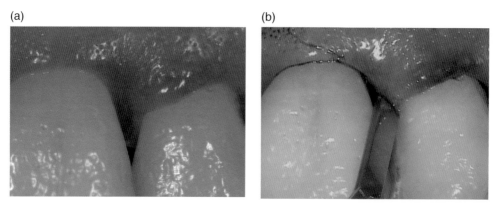

Figure 8.2   (a) The interdental space between the central and lateral incisor is narrow. (b) The microblade is positioned in the interdental space to cut a diagonal incision according to the principles of the SPPF.

(a)   (b)

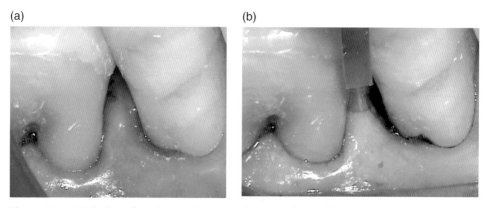

Figure 8.3   (a) The interdental space between the premolar and the molar is wide. (b) The microblade is positioned in the interdental space to cut a horizontal incision according to the principles of the MPPT.

In both the SPPF and MPPT incisions, the microblade is aimed at reaching the underlying bone: it may be necessary to run the scalpel two or three times to get a sharp separation between the buccal and the lingual interdental soft tissues.

The buccal incision is then continued in the interdental and buccal sulcus of the defect- and crest-associated teeth. The mesio-distal extension is kept to a minimum: when an isolated interdental defect is made, the incision should not invade the next interdental papillae. The lingual/palatal incision is very similar to the buccal one: care has to be taken not to damage the defect-associated papilla, keeping the microblade strictly intrasulcular.

Both the buccal and the lingual intrasulcular incisions should reach the residual bone; then, buccal and lingual full thickness flaps are elevated with tiny periosteal elevators to uncover the defect and the residual bone crest (Figure 8.4a–i). The corono-apico elevation is meant to expose 1–2 mm of bone crest: should the elevation require a greater apical extension (e.g., in cases in which the buccal or

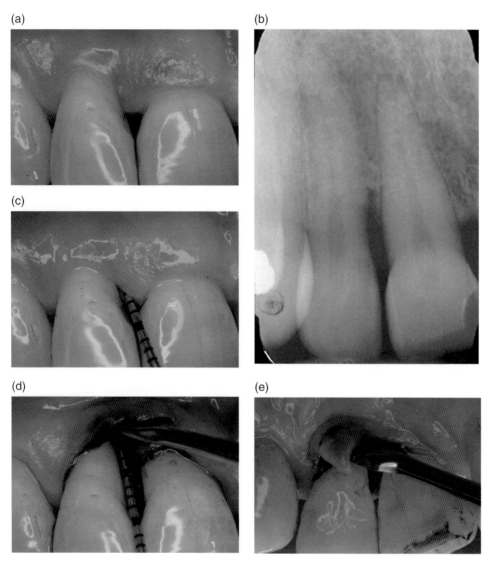

Figure 8.4   (a) Fifty-five-year-old patient presenting with chronic generalized periodontitis reported a family history for periodontitis, was systemically healthy, and a nonsmoker. After cause-related therapy, FMPS and FMBS were less than 15%, and most of the pockets were resolved. A pocket was still present at the upper right lateral incisor. (b) The radiograph shows the presence of a narrow intrabony defect associated with a suprabony component. (c) A 7 mm pocket associated with a 2 mm recession was measured at the mesial aspect of the lateral incisor. A 6 mm pocket was also detectable on the mid-palatal side. The clinical objective was to reduce the probing depth, thereby minimizing the retraction of the gingival margin. (d, e) The surgical site was approached with a MIST. The buccal flap involved the defect-associated interdental papilla and was minimally extended to the mid-buccal area of the lateral and central incisors. The interdental papilla was reflected toward the palatal side. The palatal flap was minimally elevated. A narrow 5 mm 1–2 wall intrabony defect was evident after debridement.

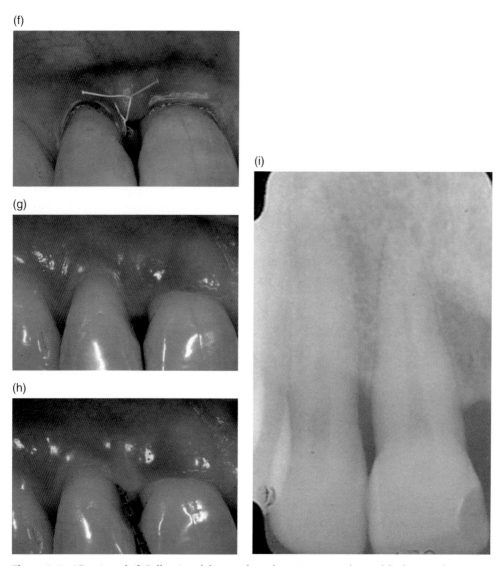

Figure 8.4 *(Continued)* (f) Following delivery of amelogenins, a single modified internal mattress suture was positioned to close the flap. (g) The 1-year photograph shows healthy condition of the treated area. (h) A 2 mm probing depth at 1 year compares with the 7 mm recorded at baseline. The gingival margin is stable. (i) The radiograph shows the resolution of the intrabony component of the defect.

lingual bone wall(s) is missing or the defect is involving an ample area of the lingual side), the flap has to be extended in mesial or distal direction to allow for a greater flap mobility (Figure 8.5a–m). In some instances, buccal and/or lingual vertical releasing incisions can be added to increase the reflection of the flaps. These additional incisions are to be performed only when necessary and are aimed at increasing the access to the defect. No split thickness incisions are used—the

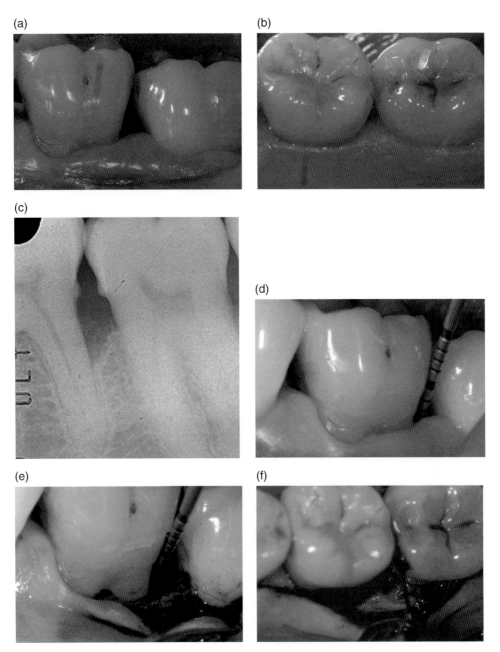

Figure 8.5 (a) A 62-year-old male presenting with chronic generalized periodontitis. He reported a family history for periodontitis, was systemically healthy and former smoker. At baseline FMPS and FMBS were over 80%. Cause-related therapy required about 3 months, after which FMPS and FMBS were reduced to less than 15%. Pockets were still present on few teeth, including the lower left first molar. (b) The radiograph, shows the presence of a 45° wide intrabony defect distal to the first molar. (c) The periodontal probe reveals a 7 mm pocket associated with 1 mm recession distal to the molar. A 6 mm pocket was also present on the distal and the mid-palatal side. The clinical objective was to reduce the probing depth. (d, e) The site was approached with a MIST. The buccal flap involved only the defect-associated interdental papilla and was extended to the mid-buccal area of the two molars. The lingual flap was extended also to the papilla between molar and premolar, to obtain proper access for defect debridement. A 6 mm three-wall intrabony defect was evident after debridement. The bone defect extended to the lingual side, reaching the mesial root of the first molar.

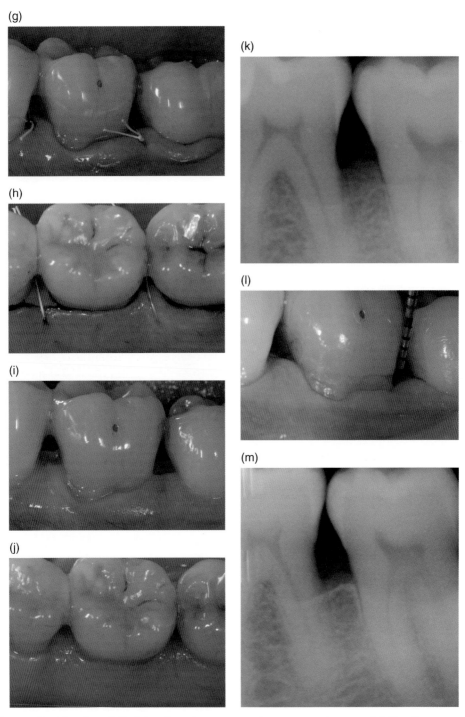

Figure 8.5 (*Continued*) (f, g) Amelogenins were used as regenerative material. The flap was sutured with a single modified internal mattress suture at the defect associated papilla. The papilla mesial to the first molar was sutured with a passing suture. (i, j) Primary closure was maintained at 1 week, when sutures were removed. (k) The 1-year radiograph shows the complete resolution of the intrabony component of the defect. (l) The 3-year photograph shows 4 mm probing depth. (m) The 3-year radiograph shows stability of the regenerated bone.

aim of flap elevation being to expose the coronal edge of the residual bone crest. In most of the cases, the reflection of the buccal flap does not involve the mucogingival junction.

When both the buccal and lingual flaps are reflected, scaling and root planing are performed by means of minicurettes and sonic/ultrasonic instruments. The aim of instrumentation is to fully remove soft tissue from the bone defect and to carefully debride and plane the root surface. Once thoroughly cleaned, the defect can be treated with different regenerative materials, such as amelogenins, growth factors, autologous bone grafts, allograft materials, or combinations thereof. Barrier membranes are not to be used in combination with the MIST: barrier placement, in fact, requires a larger extension of the flap and, frequently, a split thickness approach, according to the surgical design of the modified papilla preservation technique [7,15] and the simplified papilla preservation flap [24]. The use of amelogenins should also include the application of EDTA for 2 min on the air-dried root surface; the root surface is then thoroughly washed and gently air-dried to apply amelogenins.

The suture technique is based on the application of a single modified internal mattress suture (the use of a 6-0 PTFE suture is suggested) to provide a primary intention closure of the interdental papilla. The primary intention seal can be improved by applying additional passing sutures (the use of 6-0 or 7-0 monofilaments is suggested), when needed.

The MIST can also be used to treat multiple intrabony defects on adjacent teeth [37]. In this instance, the technique requires a mesio-distal extension of the flap to include all the defects-associated teeth and to allow for the elevation of all the defect-associated papillae. Although the mesio-distal extension is increased, the corono-apical elevation of the full thickness buccal and lingual/palatal flap is minimal, according to the previously reported principles.

Modified MIST

The M-MIST has been proposed to further reduce invasivity and patient side effects, and to increase the odds for primary closure of the wound and for blood clot stability [38]. The overall idea of the M-MIST is to provide a very small interdental access to the defect through a small buccal window (Figure 8.6a–i). The entry incision is performed on the buccal side of the interdental papilla and follows the same principles described for the MIST approach. The interdental incisions involve the buccal aspect of the teeth neighboring the defect and do not involve the next papillae. When the microblade has completed a sharp dissection of gingiva, a triangular buccal flap is minimally elevated to expose the residual buccal bone crest. Once the buccal flap has been reflected, the microblade is positioned to dissect the supracrestal interdental tissue from the granulation tissue: the blade should aim at the buccal surface of the lingual bony wall. The angulation of the blade will, therefore, be different with different bone anatomies: the more apical the lingual/palatal bone destruction, the greater the corono-apical

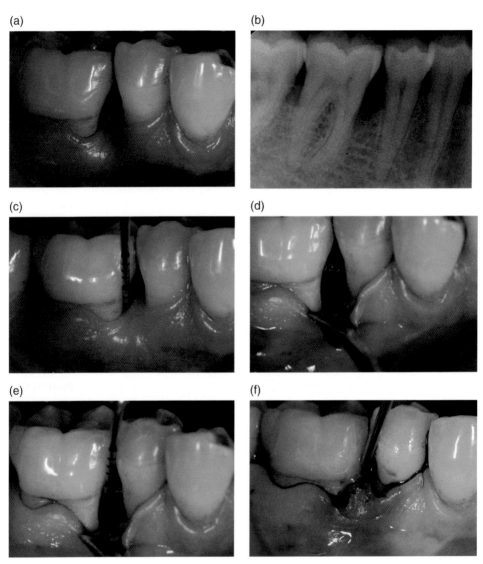

Figure 8.6 (a) A 35-year-old male presenting with aggressive localized periodontitis. He reported a family history for periodontitis, was systemically healthy, and a nonsmoker. At baseline FMPS was 30% and FMBS 58%. After cause-related therapy, FMPS and FMBS were reduced to less than 15%. A pocket was still present on the lower right first molar. (b) The radiograph shows the presence of a 40° wide intrabony defect mesial to the first molar. (c) The periodontal probe reveals a 6 mm pocket associated with 2 mm recession limited to the mesial side of the molar. The clinical objective was to reduce the probing depth. (d) The site was approached with an M-MIST. The tiny triangular buccal flap involved only the defect-associated interdental papilla and was minimally extended to the mid-area of mesial root of the molar and of the premolar. The interdental papilla was not reflected, and the lingual flap was not elevated. The granulation tissue was removed from under the papilla, and root debridement was performed through the small buccal window. (e) The three-wall intrabony defect was 6 mm deep. (f) Amelogenins were delivered into the defect.

(g)

(h)

(i)

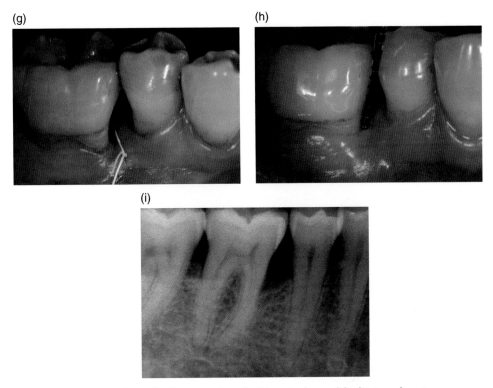

Figure 8.6 *(Continued)* (g) The flap was closed with a single modified internal mattress suture. (h) At 1 year, a probing depth of 2 mm was associated with 2 mm of gingival recession. (i) The 1-year radiograph shows the almost complete resolution of the intrabony component of the defect.

inclination of the blade. When the blade has sharply separated the papillary from the granulation tissue, the latter is removed with minicurettes. The interdental papilla is not detached from the residual interdental bone crest and supracrestal fibers, and the palatal flap is not elevated. Then, the root surface is thoroughly scaled and planed by the combined action of minicurettes and sonic/ultrasonic instruments. Special attention has to be paid to avoid any trauma to the supracrestal fibers of the defect-associated papilla. As reported for the MIST, the bone defect can be treated with different regenerative materials, such as amelogenins, growth factors, autologous bone grafts, allograft materials, or combinations thereof, but not barrier membranes.

All the reported clinical steps are performed through the small buccal "surgical window" and require magnifying devices and optimal illumination of the surgical field, such as an operative microscope or magnifying lenses. The primary closure of the surgical wound is achieved using a modified internal mattress suture and eventually the application of additional passing sutures, as described for the MIST technique (Figure 8.7a–j).

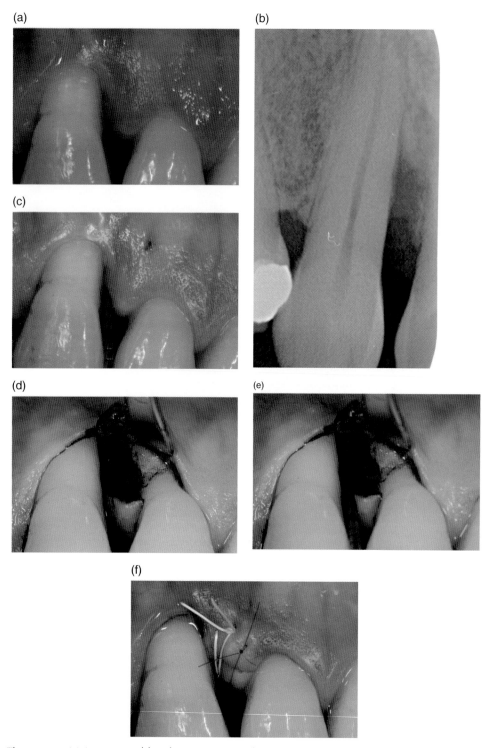

Figure 8.7 (a) A 59-year-old male presenting with chronic generalized periodontitis. He did not report a family history for periodontitis, was systemically healthy, and a former smoker. FMPS and FMBS were reduced to less than 15% after cause-related therapy. Pockets were still present on some teeth, including the upper right cuspid. (b) The radiograph shows the presence of a narrow intrabony defect mesial to the cuspid.

(g)

(h)

(j)

(i)

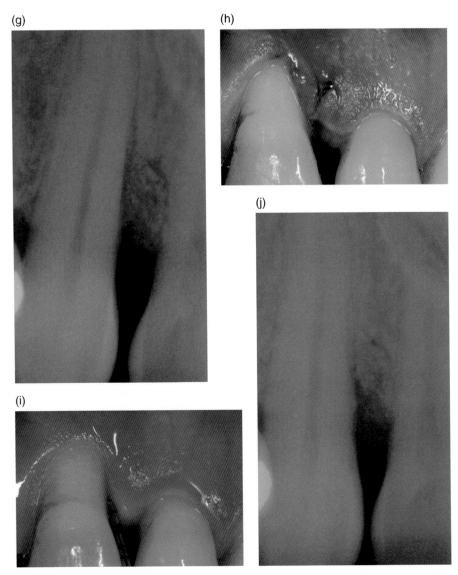

Figure 8.7 (*Continued*) (c) The periodontal probe reveals a 7 mm pocket and a consistent gingival recession. The clinical objective was to reduce the probing depth minimizing any further gingival retraction. (d) The site was approached with an M-MIST. The tiny triangular buccal flap involved only the defect-associated papilla. The interdental papilla was not reflected and the lingual flap was not elevated. After removal of the granulation tissue from under the papilla, root debridement was performed through the small buccal window. (e) A 6 mm-deep one-, two-, and three-wall intrabony defect was evident after debridement. The defect was treated with a combination of amelogenins and a filler to minimize the collapse of the papilla. (f). The flap was closed with a modified internal mattress suture and an additional passing suture. (g) The postoperative radiograph shows the presence of biomaterial filling the intrabony component of the defect. (h) Sutures were removed at 1 week. Primary closure of the flap was maintained. (i) At 1 year, probing depth was 3 mm. There was no increment of gingival recession. (j) The 1-year radiograph shows the complete resolution of the intrabony component of the defect.

Choice of the regenerative material

Selection of the regenerative material is based on the defect anatomy and on the flap design chosen to access the defect. As clearly seen from a review of the scientific literature [5], the clinical decision to implant a barrier and/or a filler takes its foundations in the need to stabilize the blood clot and the surgical flap. This becomes more necessary when treating a one-wall or a wide two-wall defect. The need for extra stabilization of the treated area increases when a large flap with high degree of mobility is designed. When treating narrow two-wall and three-wall defects, the bone anatomy *per se* provides enough stability, especially when a low-mobility, minimally invasive flap in designed. The published evidence shows that, applying the M-MIST, the flap alone without additional use of regenerative materials, the outcomes are as good as with the additional use of regenerative materials. Therefore, when approaching a site with minimally invasive surgery, a possible decisional tree is the following:

1. When an M-MIST approach is applied, amelogenins or growth factors, or no regenerative materials are the possible choices, irrespective of the bone anatomy. In other words, there is no great need for a supportive biomaterial, and most probably, there is little advantage in using regenerative substances (Figure 8.8a–d).
2. If a MIST approach is applied, amelogenins or growth factors can be used in containing defects (narrow two-wall and three-wall) or in combination with a filler in noncontaining defects (one-wall or a wide two-wall).

Technical implications

Application of MIST and M-MIST requires surgical skills and a proper surgical setting. The major problem to overcome applying minimally invasive surgery is the problem of visibility and manipulation of the surgical field, in particular, with the M-MIST approach. In fact, the minimal flap reflection reduces the angle of vision and, especially, the light penetration into the surgical field. High magnification and direct optimal illumination provided by a surgical microscope or magnifying lenses can be of great help. In addition, the soft tissue manipulation during instrumentation requires special care since the flaps, not fully reflected, lay very close to the working field. Small instruments, such as small periosteal elevators and tiny tissue forceps are mandatory as well as their gentle application to soft and hard tissues. Microblades, minicurettes, and miniscissors allow for a full control of the incision, debridement, and refinement of the surgical area, as well as sutures from 6-0 to 8-0 are requested for the wound closure.

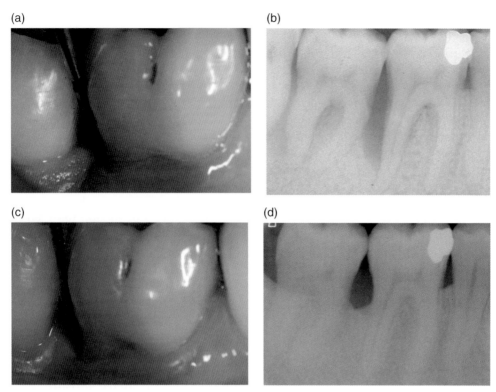

Figure 8.8   (a, b) Severe intrabony defect distal to the first lower molar, associated with a deep interproximal pocket. (c, d) Three years after regenerative therapy, the bone defect was completely resolved and the pocket eliminated. The site was treated with M-MIST alone, without any additional regenerative material.

Postsurgical protocols

Postsurgical and early home care protocols are directly taken from the experiences developed from running many controlled clinical trials [7,46–51]. An empirical protocol for the control of bacterial contamination consisting of doxicycline (100 mg bid for 1 week), 0.12% chlorhexidine mouth rinsing three times per day, and weekly prophylaxis is prescribed. Sutures are removed after 1 week. Patients are requested to avoid normal brushing, flossing, and chewing in the treated area for periods of 4–6 weeks. A postsurgical soft toothbrush soaked in chlorhexidine is used from week 1 to gently wipe the treated area. Patients can resume full oral hygiene and chewing function in the treated area 4–6 weeks after suture removal. At the end of the "early healing phase," patients are placed on periodontal maintenance every 3 months' recall system. A general suggestion to avoid any invasive clinical intervention, such as hard subgingival instrumentation, restorative dentistry, orthodontics, and additional surgery, for a period of about 9 months is also part of a strategy that is aimed at optimizing the clinical outcomes of periodontal regeneration.

Postoperative period and local side effects

From the very beginning of the "guided tissue regeneration era," it was apparent the frequent occurrence of complications, in particular, exposure of barriers. It amounted to almost 100% of the cases in the pre-papilla preservation technique period and was reportedly reduced to an amount ranging from 50% to 6% when papilla preservation flaps were adopted [5]. A consistent decrease of complications was observed when barriers were not incorporated in the surgical procedure. In particular, the adoption of amelogenins largely reduced the prevalence of complications [4,23,49].

The development of minimally invasive surgery has further reduced the amount of complications and side effects in the postoperative period.

Primary closure of the flap was reported in 100% of cases treated with MIST and maintained in 95% of the cases at 1 week in single sites [36,39] and in 100% of the cases in treatment of multiple sites [37]. Edema was noted in few cases [36,37,39]. No postsurgical hematoma, suppuration, flap dehiscence, presence of granulation tissue, or other complications were reported in any of the treated sites [36,37,39]. Root sensitivity is not a frequent occurrence. It was reported at 1 week by about 20% of the patients and rapidly decreased in the following weeks; at week 6, only one patient still reported some root sensitivity [39]. Ribeiro et al. [40] reported that the extent of root hypersensitivity, and edema was minimum, and no patients developed hematomas.

When applying the M-MIST [38], the reported primary closure was obtained and maintained in 100% of the cases. In a second controlled study [31], one M-MIST/EMD/BMDX site presented at suture removal (week 1) with a slight discontinuity of the interdental wound. At week 2, the gap appeared closed.

No edema, hematoma, or suppuration was noted in any of the treated sites [31,38].

Conclusions

Minimally invasive surgery should be considered a true reality in the field of periodontal regeneration. Cohort studies and randomized controlled clinical trials have demonstrated its potential to greatly improve the periodontal conditions of sites associated with intrabony defects, proving its efficacy. These clinical improvements are consistently associated with very limited morbidity to the patient during the surgical procedure as well as in the postoperative period. Chair-time required to perform such a surgery is by far shorter than the one required for more conventional surgical approaches. Minimally invasive surgery, however, cannot be applied at all cases. A step-wise decisional algorithm should support clinicians in choosing the proper approach.

References

1. Matuliene, G., Pjetursson, B.E., Salvi, G.E. *et al.* (2008) Influence of residual pockets on progression of periodontitis and tooth loss: Results after 11 years of maintenance. *Journal of Clinical Periodontology*, **35**, 685–695.
2. Murphy, K.G. & Gunsolley, J.C. (2003) Guided tissue regeneration for the treatment of periodontal intrabony and furcation defects. A systematic review. *Annals of Periodontology*, **8**, 266–302.
3. Needleman, I.G., Worthington, H.V., Giedrys-Leeper, E. & Tucker, R.J. (2006) Guided tissue regeneration for periodontal infra-bony defects. *Cochrane Database of Systematic Reviews*, **(2)**,CD001724. Review.
4. Esposito, M., Grusovin, M.G., Papanikolaou, N., Coulthard, P. & Worthington, H.V. (2009) Enamel matrix derivative (Emdogain) for periodontal tissue regeneration in intrabony defects. A Cochrane systematic review. *European Journal of Oral Implantology*, **2**, 247–266. Review.
5. Cortellini, P. & Tonetti, M.S. (2014) Clinical concepts for regenerative therapy in intrabony defects. *Periodontology 2000* (in press).
6. Cortellini, P., Pini-Prato, G. & Tonetti, M. (1993) Periodontal regeneration of human infrabony defects. I. Clinical measures. *Journal of Clinical Periodontology*,**64**, 254–260.
7. Cortellini, P., Pini-Prato, G. & Tonetti, M. (1995) Periodontal regeneration of human infrabony defects with titanium reinforced membranes. A controlled clinical trial. *Journal of Clinical Periodontology*, **66**, 797–803.
8. Mayfield, L., Söderholm, G., Hallström, H. *et al.* (1998) Guided tissue regeneration for the treatment of intraosseous defects using a bioabsorbable membrane. A controlled clinical study. *Journal of Clinical Periodontology*, **25**, 585–595.
9. Silvestri, M., Sartori, S., Rasperini, G., Ricci, G., Rota, C. & Cattaneo, V. (2003) Comparison of infrabony defects treated with enamel matrix derivative versus guided tissue regeneration with a nonresorbable membrane. A multicenter controlled clinical trial. *Journal of Clinical Periodontology*, **30**, 386–393.
10. Tonetti, M., Pini-Prato, G. & Cortellini, P. (1993) Periodontal regeneration of human infrabony defects. IV. Determinants of the healing response. *Journal of Periodontology*, **64**, 934–940.
11. Tonetti, M., Pini-Prato, G. & Cortellini, P. (1995) Effect of cigarette smoking on periodontal healing following GTR in infrabony defects. A preliminary retrospective study. *Journal of Clinical Periodontology*, **22**, 229–234.
12. Tonetti, M., Pini-Prato, G. & Cortellini, P. (1996) Factors affecting the healing response of intrabony defects following guided tissue regeneration and access flap surgery. *Journal of Clinical Periodontology*, **23**, 548–556.
13. Haney, J.M., Nilveus, R.E., McMillan, P.J. & Wikesjo, U.M.E. (1993) Periodontal repair in dogs: Expanded polytetrafluorethylene barrier membrane support wound stabilisation and enhance bone regeneration. *Journal of Periodontology*, **64**, 883–890.
14. Sigurdsson, T.J., Hardwick, R., Bogle, G.C. & Wikesjo, U.M.E. (1994) Periodontal repair in dogs: Space provision by reinforced ePTFE membranes enhances bone and cementum regeneration in large supraalveolar defects. *Journal of Periodontology*, **65**, 350–356.
15. Cortellini, P., Pini-Prato, G. & Tonetti, M. (1995) The modified papilla preservation technique. A new surgical approach for interproximal regenerative procedures. *Journal of Clinical Periodontology*, **66**, 261–266.

16. Wikesjo, U.M.E., Lim, W.H., Thomson, R.C., Cook, A.D. & Hardwick, W.R. (2003) Periodontal repair in dogs: Gingival tissue occlusion, a critical requirement for guided tissue regeneration. *Journal of Clinical Periodontology*, **30**, 655–664.

17. Kim, C.S., Choi, S.H., Chai, J.K. *et al.* (2004) Periodontal repair in surgically created intrabony defects in dogs. Influence of the number on bone walls on healing response. *Journal of Periodontology*, **75**, 229–235.

18. Linghorne, W.J. & O'Connel, D.C. (1950) Studies in the regeneration and reattachment of supporting structures of teeth. I. Soft tissue reattachment. *Journal of Dental Research*,**29**, 419–428.

19. Hiatt, W.H., Stallard, R.E., Butler, E.D. & Badget, B. (1968) Repair following mucoperiosteal flap surgery with full gingival retention. *Journal of Periodontology*, **39**, 11–16.

20. Wikesjo, U.M.E. & Nilveus, R. (1990) Periodontal repair in dogs: Effect of wound stabilisation on healing. *Journal of Periodontology*, **61**, 719–724.

21. Selvig, K., Kersten, B. & Wikesjö, U.M.E. (1993) Surgical treatment of intrabony periodontal defects using expanded polytetrafluoroethylene barrier membranes: Influence of defect configuration on healing response. *Journal of Periodontology*, **64**, 730–733.

22. DeSanctis, M., Clauser, C. & Zucchelli, G. (1996) Bacterial colonization of barrier material and periodontal regeneration.*Journal of Clinical Periodontology*, **23**, 1039–1046.

23. Sanz, M., Tonetti, M.S., Zabalegui, I. *et al.* (2004) Treatment of intrabony defects with enamel matrix proteins or barrier membranes: Results from a multicenter practice-based clinical trial. *Journal of Periodontology*, **75**, 726–733.

24. Cortellini, P., Pini-Prato, G. & Tonetti, M. (1999) The simplified papilla preservation flap. A novel surgical approach for the management of soft tissues in regenerative procedures.*The International Journal of Periodontics & Restorative Dentistry*,**19**, 589–599.

25. Cortellini, P. & Tonetti, M.S. Microsurgical approach to periodontal regeneration. Initial evaluation in a case cohort. *Journal of Periodontology*, **72**, 559–569.

26. Cortellini, P. & Tonetti, M.S. (2005) Clinical performance of a regenerative strategy for intrabony defects: Scientific evidence and clinical experience. *Journal of Periodontology*, **76**, 341–350.

27. Wachtel, H., Schenk, G., Bohm, S., Weng, D., Zuhr, O. & Hurzeler, M.B. (2003) Microsurgical access flap and enamel matrix derivative for the treatment of periodontal intrabony defects: A controlled clinical study. *Journal of Clinical Periodontology*, **30**, 496–504.

28. Francetti, L., Del Fabbro, M., Calace, S., Testori, T. & Weinstein, R.L. (2005) Microsurgical treatment of gingival recession: A controlled clinical study. *The International Journal of Periodontics & Restorative Dentistry*, **25**, 181–188.

29. Burkhardt, R. & Lang, N.P. (2005) Coverage of localized gingival recessions: Comparison of micro- and macrosurgical techniques. *Journal of Clinical Periodontology*, **32**, 287–293.

30. Zuhr, O., Fickl, S., Wachtel, H., Bolz, W. & Hurzeler, M.B. (2007) Covering of gingival recessions with a modified microsurgical tunnel technique: Case report. *The International Journal of Periodontics & Restorative Dentistry*, **27**, 457–463.

31. Fickl, S., Thalmair, T., Kebschull, M., Böhm, S. & Wachtel, H. (2009) Microsurgical access flap in conjunction with enamel matrix derivative for the treatment of intrabony defects: A controlled clinical trial. *Journal of Clinical Periodontology*, **36**, 784–790.

32. Cortellini, P., Tonetti, M.S. & Pini-Prato, G. (2012) The partly epithelialized free gingival graft (PE-FGG) at lower incisors. A pilot study with implications for alignment of the muco-gingival junction. *Journal of Clinical Periodontology*, **39**, 674–680.

33. Harrel, S.K. & Rees, T.D. (1995) Granulation tissue removal in routine and minimally invasive surgical procedures. *Compendium of Continuing Education Dentistry*, **16**, 960–967.

34. Harrel, S.K. & Nunn, M.E. (2001) Longitudinal comparison of the periodontal status of patients with moderate to severe periodontal disease receiving no treatment, non-surgical treatment, and surgical treatment utilizing individual sites for analysis. *Journal of Periodontology*, **72**, 1509–1519.

35. Harrel, S.K., Wilson, T.G. Jr. & Nunn, M.E. (2005) Prospective assessment of the use of enamel matrix proteins with minimally invasive surgery. *Journal of Periodontology*, **76**, 380–384.

36. Cortellini, P. & Tonetti, M.S. (2007) A minimally invasive surgical technique (MIST) with enamel matrix derivate in the regenerative treatment of intrabony defects: A novel approach to limit morbidity. *Journal of Clinical Periodontology*, **34**, 87–93.

37. Cortellini, P., Nieri, M., Pini-Prato, G.P. & Tonetti, M.S. (2008) Single minimally invasive surgical technique (MIST) with enamel matrix derivative (EMD) to treat multiple adjacent intrabony defects. Clinical outcomes and patient morbidity. *Journal of Clinical Periodontology*, **35**, 605–613.

38. Cortellini, P. & Tonetti, M.S. (2009) Improved wound stability with a modified minimally invasive surgical technique in the regenerative treatment of isolated interdental intrabony defects. *Journal of Clinical Periodontology*, **36**, 157–163.

39. Cortellini, P. & Tonetti, M.S. (2007) Minimally invasive surgical technique (M.I.S.T.) and enamel matrix derivative (EMD) in intrabony defects. (I) Clinical outcomes and intra-operative and post-operative morbidity. *Journal of Clinical Periodontology*, **34**, 1082–1088.

40. Ribeiro, F.V., Casarin, R.C., Palma, M.A., Júnior, F.H., Sallum, E.A. & Casati, M.Z. (2011) The role of enamel matrix derivative protein in minimally invasive surgery in treating intrabony defects in single rooted teeth: A randomized clinical trial. *Journal of Periodontology*, **82**, 522–532.

41. Ribeiro, F.V., Casarin, R.C., Palma, M.A., Júnior, F.H., Sallum, E.A. & Casati, M.Z. (2011) Clinical and patient-centered outcomes after minimally invasive non-surgical or surgical approaches for the treatment of intrabony defects: A randomized clinical trial. *Journal of Periodontology*, **82**, 1256–1266.

42. Cortellini, P. & Tonetti, M.S. (2011) Clinical and radiographic outcomes of the modified minimally invasive surgical technique with and without regenerative materials: A randomized-controlled trial in intra-bony defects. *Journal of Clinical Periodontology*, **38**, 365–373.

43. Trombelli, L., Simonelli, A., Pramstraller, M., Wikesjo, U.M.E. & Farina, R. (2010) Single flap approach with and without guided tissue regeneration and a hydroxyapatite biomaterial in the management of intraosseous periodontal defects. *Journal of Periodontology*, **81**, 1256–1263.

44. Mishra, A., Avula, H., Pathakota, K.R. & Avula, J. (2013) Efficacy of modified minimally invasive surgical technique in the treatment of human intrabony defects with or without use of rhPDGF-BB gel: a randomized controlled trial. *Journal of Clinical Periodontology*, **40** (2), 172–179.

45. Papapanou, P.N. & Tonetti, M. (2000) Diagnosis and epidemiology of periodontal osseous lesions. *Periodontology*, **22**, 8–21.

46. Cortellini, P., Pini-Prato, G. & Tonetti, M. (1996) Periodontal regeneration of human intrabony defects with bioresorbable membranes. A controlled clinical trial. *Journal of Clinical Periodontology*, **67**, 217–223.

47. Cortellini, P., Tonetti, M.S., Lang, N.P. *et al.* (2001) The simplified papilla preservation flap in the regenerative treatment of deep intrabony defects: Clinical outcomes and postoperative morbidity. *Journal of Periodontology*, **72**, 1701–1712.

48. Tonetti, M., Cortellini, P., Suvan, J.E. *et al.* (1998) Generalizability of the added benefits of guided tissue regeneration in the treatment of deep intrabony defects. Evaluation in a multi-center randomized controlled clinical trial. *Journal of Periodontology*, **69**, 1183–1192.

49. Tonetti, M.S., Lang, N.P., Cortellini, P. *et al.* (2002) Enamel matrix proteins in the regenerative therapy of deep intrabony defects. A multicenter randomized controlled clinical trial. *Journal of Clinical Periodontology*, **29**, 317–325.

50. Tonetti, M.S., Cortellini, P., Lang, N.P. *et al.* (2004) Clinical outcomes following treatment of human intrabony defects with GTR/bone replacement material or access flap alone. A multicenter randomized controlled clinical trial. *Journal of Clinical Periodontology*, **31**, 770–776.

51. Tonetti, M.S., Fourmousis, I., Suvan, J., Cortellini, P., Bragger, U. & Lang, N.P.; European Research Group on Periodontology (ERGOPERIO)(2004) Healing, post-operative morbidity and patient perception of outcomes following regenerative therapy of deep intrabony defects. *Journal of Clinical Periodontology*, **31**, 1092–1098.

9 Minimally Invasive Soft Tissue Grafting

Edward P. Allen and Lewis C. Cummings

Soft tissue grafting is indicated for augmenting sites with deficient-attached gingiva and for covering exposed roots. Surgical grafting techniques have evolved over the past 50 years to a minimally invasive method with refinements in recipient site preparation and the use of allograft donor tissue rather than harvesting tissue from the palate. A distinct advantage when allografts are used is that multiple teeth can be treated in one visit without concern for the amount of palatal tissue available. Regarding recipient site preparation, there has been a progression from open-site preparations to flaps with vertical incisions, to envelope flaps without vertical incisions, to tunnels with only sulcular incisions. There has also been a progression from completely exposed grafts to grafts partially covered by the recipient site flap, to grafts completely covered by coronally positioning the recipient site flap. Increased predictability of root coverage and greater patient comfort paralleled each of these advancements in recipient site design. This chapter will trace the evolution of soft tissue grafting procedures from the free gingival graft (FGG) to the current minimally invasive tunneling technique. The tunneling technique will be described in detail.

Indications for soft tissue grafting

Soft tissue grafting is indicated for augmenting the zone of attached gingiva around teeth and for covering exposed root surfaces. Attached gingiva is that portion of the gingiva that extends coronally from the mucogingival junction (MGJ) to the base of

Minimally Invasive Periodontal Therapy: Clinical Techniques and Visualization Technology, First Edition.
Edited by Stephen K. Harrel and Thomas G. Wilson Jr.
© 2015 John Wiley & Sons, Inc. Published 2015 by John Wiley & Sons, Inc.
Companion Website: www.wiley.com/go/harrel/minimallyinvasive

the gingival sulcus. It is comprised of dense collagenous connective tissue that is firmly bound down to the tooth and alveolar bone and provides a protective barrier that is resistant to the physical trauma from normal masticatory function and personal oral hygiene procedures.

A certain amount of attached gingiva is often necessary to maintain health, function, and comfort. The precise amount of attached gingiva needed varies among individuals and physical demands at the site. For example, sites where restorative margins will be placed at the gingival margin and sites where orthodontic or surgical procedures are planned might require augmentation of the attached gingiva due to the added stress of these procedures on the marginal tissue.

The vertical dimension of attached gingiva, commonly called the "width" of attached gingiva, is determined by measuring the depth of the gingival sulcus with a periodontal probe and subtracting this dimension from the vertical measurement of keratinized tissue extending from the MGJ to the mid-facial gingival crest. The thickness of the attached gingiva is also important, but its dimension is typically estimated rather than measured. In sites where there is a deficiency of attached gingiva, inflammation may be persistent, gingival recession may ensue, and the patient may experience discomfort [1]. Sites deemed to have insufficient dimensions of attached gingiva might benefit from grafting for augmentation of the gingival dimensions.

Coverage of exposed roots is another indication for soft tissue grafting, and procedures are now available to both cover roots and augment the zone of attached gingiva at the same time when indicated. Exposed roots present several patient-based problems including esthetics, root sensitivity, and increased susceptibility to cervical lesions. Complete root coverage with increased dimensions of gingiva can routinely be achieved in sites where there is no loss of interdental soft tissue or bone, thus restoring esthetics, function, and comfort [2]. In sites with loss of interdental tissues, partial root coverage can be achieved along with augmentation of gingival dimensions to resist progression of recession.

Early soft tissue grafting techniques termed free gingival grafts (FGGs) were successful in gaining an increased amount of gingiva, popularly called "gain of keratinized tissue," but required a palatal donor site consisting of both connective tissue and epithelium and were less successful for covering exposed roots. The subepithelial connective tissue graft (CTG) procedure solved the problem of root coverage and used a more comfortable internal harvest method for palatal donor tissue procurement.

The original recipient site preparation method for an FGG required creation of a vascular bed by reflecting and discarding a supraperiosteal tissue flap over the area to be grafted, while a CTG retained the reflected flap and used it to partially cover the graft. Current trends in soft tissue grafting are directed toward more minimally invasive approaches by eliminating vertical incisions and using alternatives to palatal donor tissue, both of which allow a more comfortable post operation course for the patient. The use of the tunneling technique and allograft tissue lead this trend.

Evolution of soft tissue grafting

The FGG, first described in the early 1960s [3,4], provided a means of gaining a zone of attached gingiva in sites demonstrating a gingival deficiency. This procedure was introduced during a time when the gingivectomy was a popular method for eliminating periodontal pockets, and excision of gingiva often resulted in a loss of an adequate protective zone of dense marginal gingiva. It was thought at the time that new gingiva would develop as a response to vigorous tooth brushing. In fact, minimal new marginal keratinized tissue would usually form, being derived from the periodontal ligament. The undesirable consequences of the gingivectomy were recognized and gave rise to flap procedures that preserve existing gingiva. The FGG became a widely used procedure to treat sites with surgically created deficiencies as well as to augment naturally deficient sites.

The FGG requires creation of an open vascular recipient bed and harvesting of a superficial layer of palatal donor tissue approximately 1.0–2.0 mm thick. Both epithelium and connective tissue are harvested. The donor tissue is sutured over the recipient bed, while the palatal donor site is left to heal by secondary intention. The palatal donor site is a source of discomfort and concern for the patient.

While the FGG remains the "gold standard" for gain of keratinized tissue, it was not initially a predictable procedure for coverage of deep, wide root exposure [5]. A modified FGG technique for root coverage was presented in the early 1980s [6,7]. At about the same time, the CTG method was introduced [8,9]. The harvesting of the CT graft from the palate results in an outer flap of epithelium and connective tissue that can be closed primarily, thus reducing discomfort and accelerating healing of the donor site. The CTG method has other advantages over the FGG for root coverage including greater predictability and improved esthetics. The flap created at the recipient site is retained and secured over the graft, thus providing an enhanced blood supply and improving survival of the graft over the avascular root surface. The CTG procedure is now considered to be the "gold standard" for root coverage.

Another popular root coverage technique is the coronally advanced flap (CAF), originally described in the modern era in the mid-1970s [10,11]. The CAF procedure coronally advances existing marginal gingiva to cover exposed roots without the placement of any graft. The advantages of this method include the lack of need for palatal donor tissue and enhanced esthetics. A significant limitation of the CAF is the need for adequate dimensions of gingiva apical to the exposed root surface. It is generally considered necessary to have at least 3.0 mm of gingiva vertically with a thickness of 0.8–1.0 mm to predictably cover roots [12–14].

Originally, the CAF used vertical releasing incisions. In 2000, a novel envelope flap technique with unique papillary incisions and no vertical releasing incisions was introduced [15]. This envelope flap technique has been shown to result in greater probability of complete root coverage, a better postoperative course, and better esthetics compared with a CAF with vertical incisions in the treatment of recession involving multiple adjacent teeth [16].

The CAF is used to cover CTGs where the marginal gingival dimensions are inadequate for CAF alone. As the CTG method has evolved, variations in management of the overlying tissue have been introduced. In the method originally presented by Langer and Langer, vertical incisions were used to facilitate coronal advancement of the overlying flap to partially cover the CTG [9]. Raetzke used a pouch recipient site preparation with no surface incisions but made no attempt to advance the margin coronally to cover the graft over the exposed root surface [8]. This pouch technique was limited to localized recession defects and was more successful in treating shallow recession sites than deep sites. More recently, tunnel procedures have been described for coverage of CTGs [17–20].

The tunnel technique

Currently, root coverage grafting can be accomplished with a minimally invasive tunnel technique using an allograft rather than palatal donor tissue [21,22] (Figure 9.1). Allografts have been shown to result in predictable root coverage and an increase in marginal gingival thickness equivalent to the CTG while reducing the morbidity associated with harvesting of palatal donor tissue [23–27]. A recent long-term randomized clinical trial found stability of root coverage with allografts to be equivalent to that seen with palatal CTG [28]. A distinct advantage when allografts are used is that multiple teeth can be treated in one visit without concern for the amount of palatal tissue available.

There are two separate elements to this minimally invasive soft tissue grafting technique:(i) the refined recipient site preparation and (ii) the elimination of the palatal donor site.

Recipient site preparation

The recipient site can be prepared without the need for surface incisions in treatment of most teeth with root exposure. Rather than surface incisions, intrasulcular incisions are made to release the soft tissue attachment to the cervical area of the tooth, and internal supraperiosteal sharp dissection to mobilize the pouch. The intrasulcular incisions extend from the base of the sulcus to the alveolar crest, a distance of approximately 2.0 mm comprised of the epithelial and connective tissue attachments to the root. This soft tissue attachment is often called the "biologic width," and it may extend more than the usual 2.0 mm where there is a longer connective tissue attachment due to the presence of a bony dehiscence [29]. Through this intrasulcular incision, there is access for dissection of the recipient vascular bed. The dissection extends both apically and laterally both to prepare the recipient vascular bed and to mobilize the pouch sufficiently to allow passive coronal advancement to completely cover the graft. It is necessary to extend the dissection laterally under the papillae adjacent to the treated tooth and additionally to include one tooth on either side of the tooth or teeth with

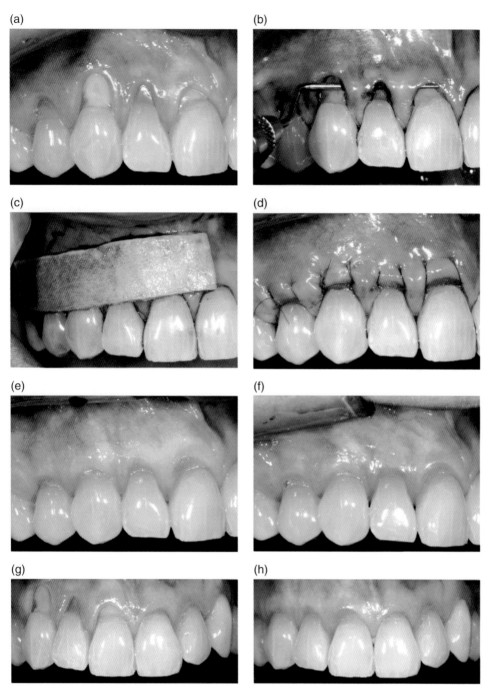

Figure 9.1 (a) Multiple tooth recession and root abrasion in the maxillary arch. (b) A tunnel site preparation has been completed. (c) The allograft on the surface before placement within the pouch. (d) The allograft and pouch were advanced together and secured at the cementoenamel junction with a 6-0 polypropylene continuous sling suture. An additional sling suture was placed around the canine for stabilization. (e) Thick marginal tissue with complete root coverage at 1 year post surgery. The patient elected not to restore the minor cervical enamel defects. (f) Maintenance of root coverage at 2 years post surgery. (g) Esthetically unappealing pretreatment appearance. (h) Improved esthetics at 8 months post surgery.

(a)
(b)
(c)
(d)

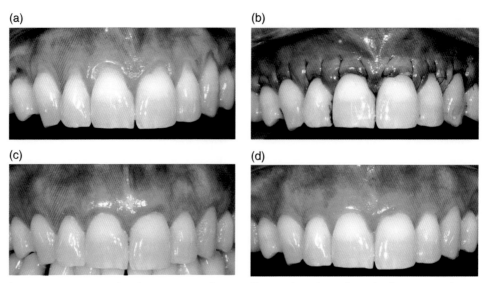

Figure 9.2 (a) Generalized recession in the maxillary arch with moderately deep cervical defects. (b) Allograft in tunnel over 7 teeth sutured with a 6-0 polypropylene continuous sling suture. An additional sling suture was placed around the left lateral incisor to stabilize the papillae. (c) Complete root coverage and thickened marginal tissue immediately following suture removal at 3 months post surgery. (d) Complete root coverage with a pleasing appearance of the gingiva that shows no evidence of surgical intervention at 2 years post surgery.

recession. This tunneling under the papillae and lateral extension of the pouch facilitate the passive coronal advancement of the pouch, thus eliminating the need for vertical releasing incisions as well as papillary incisions.

This type of site preparation is ideally suited for treating root exposure in the maxillary arch where the anatomic environment is typically favorable (Figure 9.2). There are few anatomical obstacles to interfere with the dissection process and the quality of the marginal tissue is usually better than that in the mandibular arch.

Adequate interdental embrasure space is necessary to maintain intact papillae in the tunneling process. Sites with close root approximation are subject to separation of the papillae due to a weak connection between the facial and palatal papillae. This problem is more commonly seen in the mandibular anterior region. In the mandibular arch, caution must be exercised when dissecting near the mental foramen located apical to the second premolar. There are no significant vital structures encountered when dissecting facial to the maxillary teeth.

A shallow vestibule, aberrant frenal attachments, thin tissue, bony undercuts, and an irregular alveolar bony topography represent problems to be managed when performing the tunnel technique. While all of these problems can be overcome, advanced surgical experience is required for successful outcomes, and treatment of sites with these conditions may be best left to periodontists who routinely treat such sites.

Indications for papillary incisions

The tunneling technique can be used to augment sites without recession but with minimal attached gingiva, that may be subject to developing recession. These sites include teeth that will have orthodontic treatment or restorations placed at the gingival margin. In sites with very thin tissue and no root exposure, the intrasulcular site preparation method is difficult, especially in the mandibular anterior region where the root width, and thus the sulcular width, is small. In these sites, a papillary releasing incision provides the greater access needed for dissection and graft placement (Figure 9.3). Papillary incisions should be limited to the papilla between the canine and lateral incisor when treating the mandibular anterior region. This will provide access to tunnel under the remaining papillae that will act to prevent apical retraction of the pouch and contribute to wound stability. By retaining all three papillae in the midline, the stress of muscle pull in the midline is distributed to three papillae and the likelihood of a single weak papilla tearing is reduced.

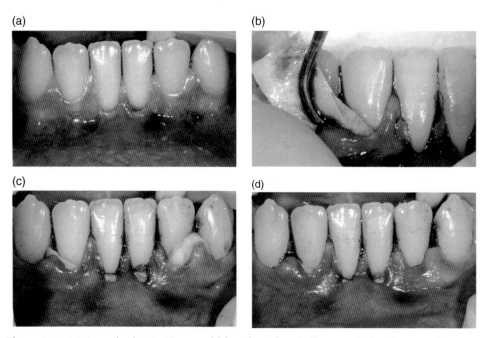

Figure 9.3 (a) Pre-orthodontic 12-year-old female with a shallow vestibule, absence of attached gingiva facial to her mandibular incisors, and thin attached gingiva facial to her lateral incisors. This site will be treated by augmentation grafting to gain a zone of dense connective tissue and deepen the vestibule. (b) A tunnel recipient site was prepared facial to all four incisors with bilateral papillary incisions between the canines and lateral incisors and an allograft was inserted through the right papillary opening. (c) The allograft was passed through the tunnel until reaching the left papillary opening. (d) The coronal border of the allograft was aligned level with the cementoenamel junction in preparation for suturing.

(e)

(f)

(g)

(h)

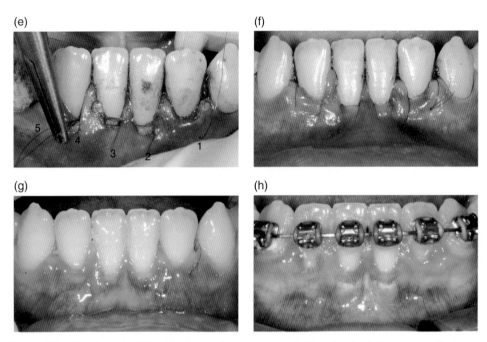

Figure 9.3 (*Continued*) (e) A continuous sling suture was initiated at the left open papilla by penetrating both the papilla and graft (1), passing through the distal embrasure and around the lingual aspect of the lateral incisor before returning to the facial through the mesial embrasure. The needle is then passed under the papilla before engaging the pouch and graft at the distal root line angle of the central incisor (2) and passing through the distal embrasure, around the lingual aspect, and back through the mesial embrasure to the facial. The needle is passed under the papilla before engaging the pouch and graft at the mesial root line angle of the right central incisor (3) and passing through the embrasure, around the lingual back to the facial, and under the papilla before engaging the pouch and graft at the mesial root line angle of the right lateral incisor (4). After passing through the mesial embrasure, around the lingual and back to the facial through the distal embrasure, the pouch and graft are engaged at the distal of the lateral incisor. The needle is then passed through the distal embrasure, around the lingual and back to the facial through the mesial embrasure. The needle is passed under the papilla (5) prior to engaging the pouch at the distal of the central incisor. (f) The continuous sling suturing sequence is continued until reaching the starting point where the suture is tied (1). (g) At 2 weeks post surgery, there is minimal edema and erythema, and the suture has disappeared into the tissue leaving only the knot exposed. There is a gain of vestibular depth and an augmentation of the marginal tissue with a dense, bound-down connective tissue beneath the mucosal surface. (h) At 30 months post surgery and near the completion of orthodontic therapy, the soft tissue has remained stable.

The advantages of eliminating vertical incisions in the tunnel recipient site preparation technique include greater degree of root coverage, better postoperative course, and better esthetics [16]. The tunnel technique was also found to result in a better postoperative course compared withan envelope flap without vertical incisions but with papillary incisions [30]. The disadvantages of the tunnel technique include the greater technical difficulty, especially in presence of the limitations described earlier. Most of the difficulty is overcome with surgical experience and the judicious use of papillary incisions where needed.

Allograft donor tissue

The second major feature of minimally invasive soft tissue grafting is the elimination of the palatal donor site. The tunnel technique provides a minimally invasive site preparation method suitable for either autologous or allogeneic donor tissue and may be used without a donor as a coronally advanced pouch in Miller Class 1 recession sites with adequate dimensions of attached gingiva [12,13]. The substitution of an allograft in place of a palatal donor provides additional advantages in soft tissue grafting. The most obvious advantage is the reduction of postoperative morbidity, potential side effects, and inconvenience for the patient associated with palatal donor surgery [31,32]. Even though the discomfort associated with palatal harvesting is greatly reduced in the CTG technique, some patients postpone or decline the needed soft tissue grafting procedure because of a perception of potential postoperative pain. Discussing with the patient that no palatal tissue will be used helps to allay much of their apprehension. The use of allograft donor tissue provides an unlimited amount of tissue for treatment of multiple teeth and sites in one surgical appointment. The palate provides a finite amount of donor tissue that varies among patients and limits the amount of soft tissue grafting that can be accomplished. This donor tissue limitation factors into treatment planning and reduces treatment to those teeth with greatest need or may require multiple surgical appointments, either of which are compromises. The use of an allograft also reduces surgical time associated with harvesting the palate. Autologous tissue may be selected for treatment of single tooth recession sites requiring minimal palatal harvesting or for sites where graft survival is compromised and the forgiving nature of autologous donor tissue is advantageous.

The most common allograft used today is an acellular dermal matrix (ADM). Of all the ADM options available today, the authors prefer AlloDerm®. Introduced in 1994 for treatment of burn patients, AlloDerm was subsequently used for additional general surgical applications as well as intra-oral soft tissue grafting procedures [33]. Since its introduction, numerous studies of AlloDerm use have been published in both the medical and the dental literature. The dental studies include RCTs, systematic reviews, and meta-analyses [23–28,31,34–38]. No other ADM has such an extensive body of scientific study and long-term history of safety and successful outcomes.

When compared to CTG, AlloDerm has been shown to result in equivalent root coverage, increase in tissue thickness, and gain of keratinized tissue [24–27,36]. Other ADM graft materials have recently become available, but they do not have the long-term positive outcomes studies of AlloDerm.

Typically, gain of keratinized tissue is minimal with a submerged grafting technique whether an allograft or a CTG is used [25–27,31]. Because of this, gain of keratinized tissue is probably not the best parameter of success for submerged grafts (Figures 9.4 and 9.5). While gain of keratinized tissue is useful for assessing graft success for surface grafts such as a free gingival graft, the amount

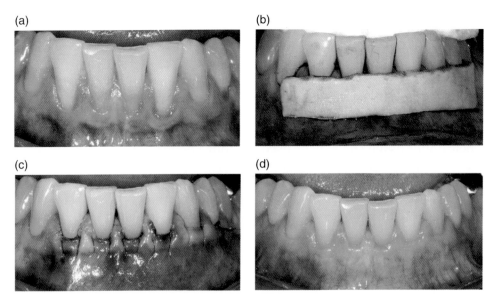

Figure 9.4 (a) Generalized recession in the mandibular anterior region with cervical notching of the left first premolar. (b) Allograft on the surface before placement in the pouch. (c) Allograft within the pouch coronally advanced with a single 6-0 polypropylene continuous sling suture. (d) Nearly complete root coverage and thickened bound-down connective tissue at 1 year post surgery.

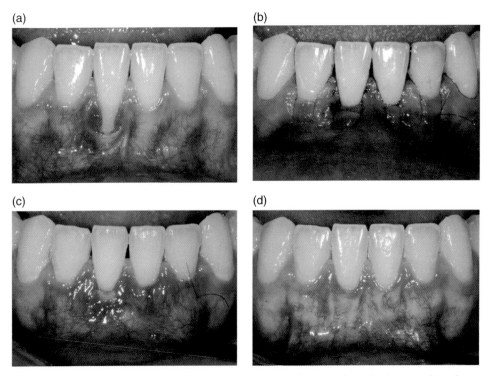

Figure 9.5 (a) Mandibular incisor with 4 mm recession, absence of attached gingival, and painful, irritated marginal tissue. The gingiva facial to the other incisors is thin. (b) Using the tunnel technique, an allograft is placed facial to all four incisors and secured with a single 6–0 polypropylene continuous sling suture. (c) At 2 weeks post surgery, the coronal border of the allograft is visible at the right central incisor. (d) At 1 year post surgery, there is complete root coverage. The thin mucosal surface belies the presence of the thick layer of dense connective tissue beneath the surface.

of keratinized tissue on the surface is not reflective of the gain of functional, dense collagenous connective tissue with submerged grafts. The small gain of keratinized tissue following a submerged grafting technique is reflective of initial graft exposure and secondary retraction of the overlying tissue exposing a small portion of the graft, and it is not an indicator of graft success.

Surgical procedure

Intrasulcular site preparation

The key feature of the tunnel technique is the elimination of traditional surface incisions and flap reflection. The recipient site is prepared by entry through the sulcus to create a pouch facial to the tooth or teeth to be treated. If multiple adjacent teeth are treated, tunneling under the papillae connects the pouches created facial to each tooth. An allograft is trimmed to size and placed within the pouch, and the graft and pouch are coronally advanced to completely cover the exposed root.

The site preparation begins with an intrasulcular incision made from the base of the sulcus to the alveolar crest using an End-Cutting Intrasulcular Knife (Hu-Friedy, Chicago, IL) (Figure 9.6b). This incision should extend horizontally from the mesiolingual line angle to the distolingual line angle of each tooth to be treated as well as one additional tooth mesial and distal to these teeth. This initial incision provides access for subperiosteal blunt reflection with an Allen Microsurgical Elevator (Hu-Friedy, Chicago, IL) (Figure 9.6c). The blunt reflection should extend laterally under the facial aspect of the papillae and apically approximately 3.0 mm past the MGJ and any bony undercuts. The papillae are elevated from the interdental crest with a Younger-Good 7/8 curette (Figure 9.6d).

Root preparation

Root preparation is performed with curettes and/or an ultrasonic instrument with a safe-sided diamond tip (Varios 750, Brasseler USA, Savannah, GA) after mobilization of the marginal tissue to allow removal of shallow restorations, elimination of angular portions of cervical lesion, and creation of a uniform root surface without damaging the soft tissue (Figure 9.6e). EDTA is applied to the root surface to remove the smear layer. The next step is apical extension and mobilization of the pouch by sharp dissection using a Modified Orban Knife (Hu-Friedy, Chicago, IL) (Figure 9.6f and g). This instrument will allow dissection that is immediately supraperiosteal to ensure passive advancement of the pouch to the CEJ and to create the required space for the graft while maintaining an immobile alveolar recipient bed.

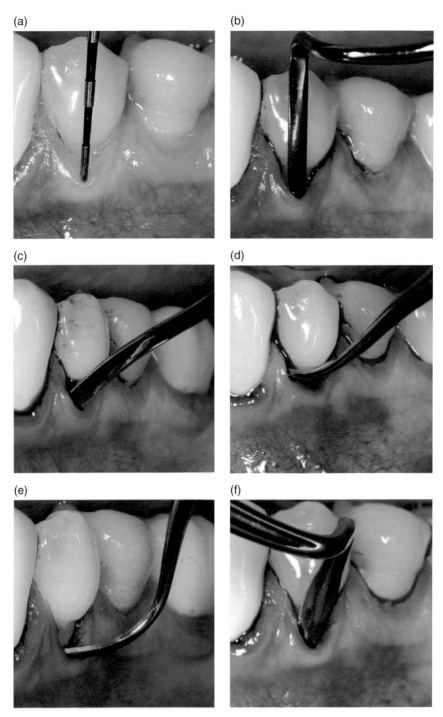

Figure 9.6 MIS technique. (a) A 3-mm root exposure with minimal marginal gingiva. (b) An incision is placed within the sulcus to detach the soft tissue from the root surface from the base of the sulcus to the alveolar crest. This incision extends from the mesiopalatal line angle around the facial aspect to the distopalatal line angle. (c) A microsurgical periosteal elevator is used to prepare a full thickness pouch under the mesial and distal papillae and facial to the root. This subperiosteal dissection extends apical to the mucogingival junction and past any bony undercuts. (d) Each papilla is elevated from the interdental alveolar crest by using a curette as a curved periosteal elevator. (e) After mobilization of the marginal tissue, the root is planed to remove any microbial deposits, sharp angles, and surface irregularities. (f) The pouch is extended apically and laterally by sharp dissection immediately supraperiosteally to allow passive coronal advancement of the pouch margin.

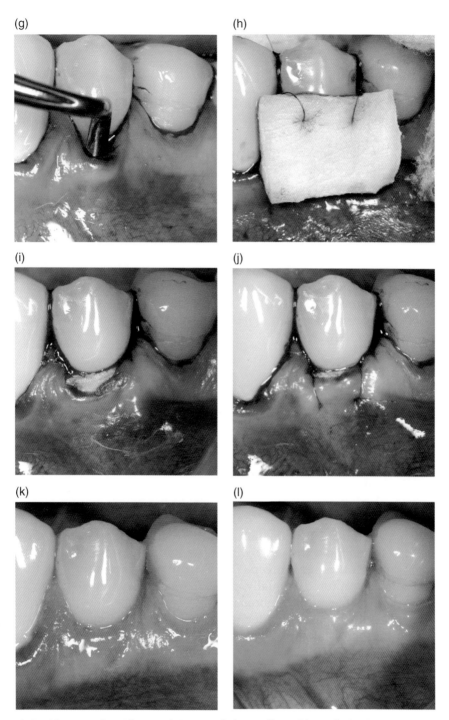

Figure 9.6 (*Continued*) (g) The pouch is extended apically and laterally by sharp dissection immediately supraperiosteally to allow passive coronal advancement of the pouch margin. (h) The allograft is trimmed to extend completely under the papillae adjacent to the exposed root. A suture may be used to aid in positioning the graft after insertion. (i) The allograft is inserted in the pouch over the root. (j) The allograft is aligned with the pouch margin and advanced together to the cementoenamel junction with a 6-0 polypropylene sling suture. (k) Complete root coverage with a thickened margin and gain of keratinized tissue is seen at 3 months post surgery. (l) Complete root coverage maintained at 2 years post surgery.

Allograft placement

The allograft is reconstituted according to the tissue bank instructions and trimmed to the proper dimensions to extend horizontally completely under the papillae mesial and distal to the treated teeth and vertically 6–8 mm (Figure 9.6h). The allograft is then soaked in a platelet-rich plasma preparation for enrichment with growth factors. The graft is inserted into the pouch through the largest sulcular opening with a Younger-Good 7/8 curette and/or by using a suture to aid insertion and positioning within the pouch (Figure 9.6i). The graft is aligned level with the gingival margins of the pouch so that both the graft and pouch may be advanced simultaneously with either a series of interrupted sling sutures or a single subpapillary continuous sling suture (Figure 9.6j) [39]. The continuous sling suture has the advantage of a single knot that is less irritating to the tissue and for the patient than multiple knots. A small diameter monofilament, nonresorbable 6-0 polypropylene suture with aC-17 needle (Hu-Friedy, Chicago, IL) is used to reduce tissue irritation and provide a longer period of stabilization.

Suturing

The continuous sling suture engages the pouch and graft at the distal aspect of each tooth progressing from the posterior toward the anterior, and then engages the pouch and graft at the mesial aspect when returning to the posterior starting point (Figure 9.3).

Beginning at the posterior-most tooth, the needle is placed through the pouch margin and allograft at a point 3.0 mm apical to the pouch margin at the distal root line angle using a microsurgical Castroviejo Needle Holder (Hu-Friedy, Chicago, IL). The microsurgical Allen Elevator (Hu-Friedy) is used at the pouch margin to help maintain the graft within the pouch. The needle is recaptured with microsurgical Dressing Forceps (Hu-Friedy) and passed through the distal embrasure space, captured lingually, passed around the lingual and back to the facial side through the mesial embrasure.

The needle is then passed under the papilla from the mesial aspect of the initial tooth to the distal aspect of the adjacent tooth. The pouch margin and graft are penetrated at the distal root line angle of the second tooth 3.0 mm apical to the pouch margin. The needle is passed back through the distal embrasure, around the tooth lingually, and then passed back to the facial side through the mesial embrasure. The needle is next passed under the papilla facially from the distal to mesial aspect, and the process continues until the last tooth to be treated is reached.

After the needle is passed around the lingual aspect of the final tooth and back through the mesial embrasure to the facial side, the pouch margin and graft are penetrated at the mesial root line angle 3.0 mm apical to the pouch margin. The needle is passed back through the mesial embrasure to the lingual side, around the tooth, and through the distal embrasure to the facial side. After passing under the papilla, the needle penetrates the pouch margin and the graft at the mesial root line angle of the next tooth, passes through the mesial embrasure, around the lingual side of the tooth, and back to the facial side through the distal embrasure. The process continues by passing under the papillae to engage the mesial root line angles of all treated teeth and finally returning to the distofacial aspect of the posterior-most tooth (starting point), to tie the suture. The surgical site is then inspected for adaptation and stability. An additional interrupted suture may be necessary on occasion for enhancement of adaptation or stabilization.

The continuous sling suture may be removed easily after swelling has subsided. Based on clinical observation, it is recommended that the suture be retained for up to 2 months to allow time for graft integration and marginal stability.

Postoperative care

The most significant postsurgical side effects are swelling and infection. Uneventful healing is facilitated by measures taken to minimize swelling. During the first 24 hours after surgery, the patient should remain inactive at home, apply ice to the face opposite the grafted site during the waking hours, have cold liquids for meals, and avoid toothbrushing. After 24 hours, the patient may return to routine nonstrenuous activities and begin eating soft foods, but should avoid mastication, tooth brushing at the surgical site, and exercise for 2 weeks. A broad-spectrum antibiotic such as Amoxicillin for 10 days post surgery and the use of an antimicrobial mouthrinse are recommended to prevent infection. A glucocorticoid such as prednisone is beneficial in reducing swelling, especially when treating multiple teeth in the mandibular arch. Pain from this procedure is usually of short duration and is managed with the usual medications.

Advantages of MI soft tissue grafting

The advantages of this minimally invasive grafting technique include(i) no surface incisions, thus no scarring; (ii) use of an allograft, which eliminates need for a palatal donor site; (iii) reduced patient discomfort; (iv) greater acceptance of treatment; and (v) ideal esthetics.

Palatal grafts are also very effective for predictable root coverage; however, they are subject to enlarging, thereby negatively impacting the esthetic outcome. Graft enlargement may be desirable in some alveolar ridge or papilla augmentation procedures, thus palatal connective tissue may be a better choice for these applications. In sites where the graft cannot be completely covered, palatal tissue will survive better than an allograft. Otherwise, an allograft is the better choice.

Application of the tunnel concept for ridge augmentation

The tunneling technique, primarily used to treat patients with gingival recession on the facial root surfaces can also be used to treat alveolar ridge defects
with rotated autogenous palatal connective tissue grafts. The rotated palatal
pedicle graft technique described by Sclar as the Vascularized Interpositional
Periosteal-Connective Tissue Graft (VIP-CT) is moderately invasive in the
approach to both graft harvest and graft placement [40]. By applying the
tunneling principles, the original technique has been modified to a less invasive grafting method to treat soft tissue defects at dental implant sites in
the esthetic zone. The less invasive nature of this procedure as compared with-
the original VIP-CT reduces postoperative complications while enhancing the
overall esthetic outcome.

The original VIP-CT grafting technique had two significant postoperative
complications: (i) palatal sloughing at the donor site and (ii) incision line opening
at the recipient site. By applying principles of minimally invasive surgery that
include remote incisions and tunneling, both of these initial complications have
been greatly reduced.

The traditional VIP-CT graft utilized a palatal incision for graft harvest located
several millimeters away from the free gingival margin. Due to the sloping position of the incision away from a fixed structure, primary closure after graft
harvest is often difficult. A lack of primary closure may result in delayed healing
and increased patient discomfort. It has been the author's experience that
beginning the palatal dissection with sulcular incisions and creation of a full-
thickness palatal envelope flap provides better access to the underlying
connective tissues for harvesting (Figure 9.7). Not only is the surgeon's ability to
dissect free periosteum and connective tissue layers improved, but the envelope
flap design allows for precise re-approximation of the flap margins to the
original incision point when harvest is complete. Securing the flap margin to
the adjacent teeth with sling sutures is adequate for incision line closing. Since
the flap has been designed as a full-thickness flap with primary closure, postoperative opening is dramatically reduced. In addition, improved visibility of the
harvest site facilitates maintenance of uniform thickness of the harvested tissue.
This better control reduces the likelihood of overthinning the palatal tissues or
perforating the epithelial layer; two common causes of postoperative palatal
discomfort and sloughing.

In addition, the original technique consisted of reflection of a facial flap to prepare the recipient site. This preparation included vertical incisions on the mesial
and distal of the defect to facilitate surgical access. These vertical incisions
increase the risk of postoperative graft exposure. In the modified version, the
recipient site is prepared by creating a pouch through remote sulcular incisions
without any vertical incisions. To maintain the integrity of the papilla on the
mesial and distal of the surgical site, which is often an implant with delicate
papilla, tunneling under the papilla and lifting them, rather than incising through
them, is performed.

(a)   (b)

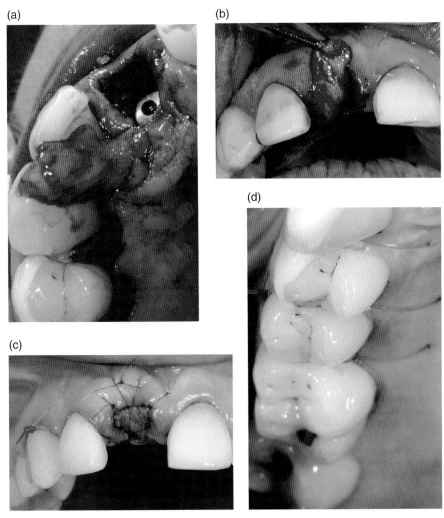

(d)

(c)

Figure 9.7   (a) Pediculated palatal connective tissue graft harvested from full flap approach. for rotation through tunnel over the coronal and facial aspects of the implant. (b) Rotation of graft before inserting through tunnel over the coronal and facial aspects of the implant. (c) Graft secured in pouch with interrupted 6–0 polypropylene sutures. (d) Primary closure of palatal donor site with

Tunneling under papillary areas and the edentulous ridge areas provides enhanced maintenance of blood supply in the surgical area. Using microsurgical instruments facilitates recipient site preparation and placement of the graft. Wound closure is accomplished with 6-0 or 7-0 sutures.

This minimally invasive technique works well for augmenting soft tissue at implant sites, especially where the ridge deficiency has a vertical component and is associated with proximal recession involving the adjacent teeth (Figure 9.8). It is especially beneficial for anterior implant sites where esthetics is often compromised due to loss of soft tissue. Indications include

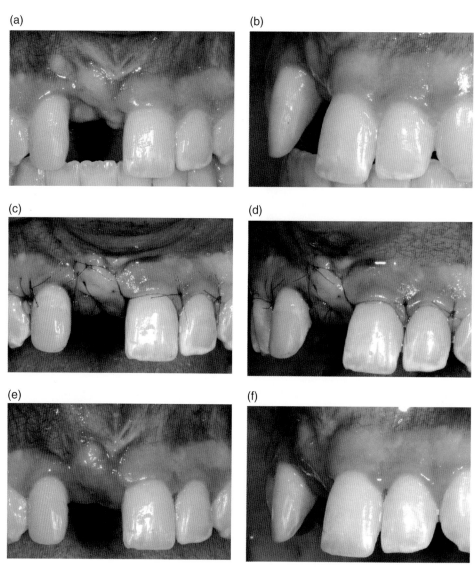

Figure 9.8   (a) (i) An alveolar ridge defect associated with facial and proximal recession on the adjacent lateral incisor in a 17-year-old female following removal of an ankylosed tooth. The site has previously been treated by bone grafting and free connective tissue grafting on separate occasions. (ii) Recession and ridge defect from the lateral aspect. (b) (i) The site was retreated with a pediculated connective tissue graft from the right palate, rotated and inserted in a tunnel created under the soft tissue over the ridge crest and facial to the lateral incisor. Papillary incisions were made distal to the right lateral incisor and left central and lateral incisors to facilitate creation of the tunnel. No vertical releasing incisions were made. The site was closed and stabilized with 6–0 polypropylene sutures. (ii) Ridge augmentation and root coverage from the lateral aspect. (c) (i and ii) Complete root coverage and ridge augmentation at 1 month post surgery. (d) (i and ii) Stability of outcome at 2 months post surgery.

(g)   (h)

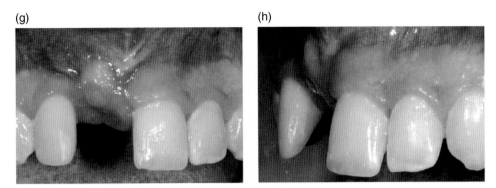

Figure 9.8   *(Continued)*

augmentation of soft tissue deficiencies at edentulous sites, augmentation during immediate implant placement, and augmentation of soft tissue deficiencies at existing implant sites

Summary

Soft tissue grafting techniques have advanced from effective but invasive methods requiring vertical releasing incisions and palatal donor tissue to current minimally invasive tunnel recipient site preparation and the use of allografts rather than palatal donor tissue. No surface incisions are required as the access for recipient site preparation is through the sulcus. This refinement in technique using microsurgical instruments and nonirritating 6-0 and 7-0 monofilament suture has resulted in a more comfortable and less intimidating procedure and postsurgical period for the patient while enhancing the esthetics of the outcome and allowing the treatment of multiple teeth in a single surgical appointment.

References

1. Lang, N.P. & Löe, H. (1972) The relationship between the width of keratinized gingiva and gingival health. *Journal of Periodontology*, **45**, 623.
2. Miller, P.D. (1985) A classification of marginal tissue recession. *The International Journal of Periodontics & Restorative Dentistry*, **5**(2), 8–13.
3. Björn, H. (1963) Free transplantation of gingiva propria. *SverigesTandlakarforbrinds Tidning*, **22**, 684–689.
4. King, K. & Pennel, B.M. (1964) *Evaluation of attempts to increase the width of attached gingiva.* Presented to the Philadelphia Society of Periodontology, April1964.
5. Sullivan, H.C. & Atkins, J.H. (1968) Free autogenous gingival grafts. I. Principles of successful grafting. *Periodontics*, **6**, 121–129.
6. Miller, P.D. (1982). Root coverage using the free soft tissue autograft following citric acid application. Part I. Technique. *The International Journal of Periodontics & Restorative Dentistry*, **2**, 64–70.

7. Miller, P.D. (1985). Root coverage using the free soft tissue autograft following citric acid application. Part III. A successful and predictable procedure in areas of deep-wide recession. *The International Journal of Periodontics & Restorative Dentistry*, **5**, 14–37.

8. Raetzke, P.B. (1985) Covering localized areas of root exposure employing the "envelope" technique. *Journal of Periodontology*, **56**, 397–402.

9. Langer, B. & Langer, L. (1985) Subepithelial connective tissue graft technique for root coverage. *Journal of Periodontology*, **56**, 715–720.

10. Restrepo, O.J. (1973) Coronally repositioned flap: Report of four cases. *Journal of Periodontology*, **44**, 564.

11. Bernimoulin, J.P., Luscher, B.&Muhlemann, H.R. (1975) Coronally repositioned flap. Clinical evaluation after one year. *Journal of Clinical Periodontology*, **2**, 1–13.

12. Allen, E.P.&Miller, P.D. (1989) Coronal positioning of existing gingiva: Short-term results in the treatment of shallow marginal tissue recession. *Journal of Clinical Periodontology*, **60**, 316–319.

13. Baldi, C., Pini-Prato, G., Pagliaro, U. *et al.*(1999) Coronally advanced flap procedure for root coverage. Is flap thickness a relevant predictor to achieve root coverage? A 19-case series. *Journal of Periodontology*, **70**, 1077–1084.

14. Huang, L.-H., Neiva, R.E.F. & Wang, H-L. (2005) Factors affecting the outcomes of coronally advanced flap root coverage procedure. *Journal of Periodontology*, **76**, 1729–1734.

15. Zucchelli, G.&De Sanctis, M. (2000) Treatment of multiple recession type defects in patients with aesthetic demands. *Journal of Periodontology*, **71**, 1506–1514.

16. Zuccheli, G., Mele, M., Mazzotti, C., Marzadori, M., Montebugnoli, L. & De Sanctis, M. (2009) Coronally advanced flap with and without vertical releasing incisions for the treatment of multiple gingival recessions: A comparative controlled randomized clinical trial. *Journal of Periodontology*, **80**, 1083–1094.

17. Allen, A.L. (1994) Use of the supraperiosteal envelope in soft tissue grafting for root coverage. I. Rationale and technique. *The International Journal of Periodontics & Restorative Dentistry*, **14**, 216–227.

18. Azzi, R. & Etienne, D. (1998) Recouvrementradiculaireet reconstruction papillaire par greffon con-jonctifenfoui sous un lambeauvestibulairetunnellisé et tractécoro-nairement. *Journal of Parodontal Implant Orale*, **17**, 71–77.

19. Blanes, R.J. & Allen, E.P. (1999) The bilateral pedicle flap-tunnel technique: A new approach to cover connective tissue grafts. *The International Journal of Periodontics & Restorative Dentistry*, **19**, 471–479.

20. Allen, E.P. (2004) Multiple tooth recession: Papilla retention pouch procedure. In: E.P. Allen (ed), *Contemporary Oral Plastic Surgery Procedural Manual*, pp. 9–16. Center for Advanced Dental Education, Dallas, TX.

21. Allen, E.P. & Cummings, L.C. (2005) Esthetics and regeneration: Acellular dermal matrix (AlloDerm). In: H. Yoshie & Y. Miyamoto (eds),*Technique and Science of Regeneration*, pp. 124–131. Quintessence, Tokyo, Japan.

22. Allen, E.P. (2006) AlloDerm: An effective alternative to palatal donor tissue for treatment of gingival recession. *Dentistry Today*, **25**, 48, 50–52.

23. Harris, R.J. (2000) A comparative study of root coverage obtained with an acellular dermal matrix versus a connective tissue graft: Results of 107 recession defects in 50 consecutively treated patients. *The International Journal of Periodontics & Restorative Dentistry*, **20**, 51–59.

24. Aichelmann-Reidy, M.E., Yukna, R.A., Evans, G.H., Nasr, H.F. & Mayer, E.T. (2001) Clinical evaluation of acellular allograft dermis for the treatment of human gingival recession. *Journal of Periodontology*, **72**, 998–1005.
25. Novaes, A.B. Jr., Grisi, D.C., Molina, G.O., Souza, S.L., Taba, M. Jr.&Grisi, M.F. (2001) Comparative 6-month clinical study of a subepithelial connective tissue graft and acellular dermal matrix graft for the treatment of gingival recession. *Journal of Periodontology*, **72**, 1477–1484.
26. Oates, T.W., Robinson, M. & Gunsolley, J.C. (2003) Surgical therapies for treatment of gingival recession. A systematic review. *Annals of Periodontology*, **8**, 303–320.
27. Gapski, R., Satheesh, K. & Wang, H.-L. (2005) Acellular dermal matrix for mucogingival surgery: A meta-analysis. *Journal of Periodontology*, **76**, 1814–1822.
28. Moslemi, N., Zazi, M.M., Haghighati, F., Morovati, S.P. & Jamali, R. (2011) Acellular dermal matrix allograft versus subepithelial connective tissue graft in treatment of gingival recessions: A 5-year randomized clinical study. *Journal of Clinical Periodontology*, **38**, 1122–1129.
29. Gargiulo, A.W., Wentz, F.M. & Orban, B. (1961) Dimensions and relations of the dento-gingival junction in humans. *Journal of Periodontology*, **32**, 261–267.
30. Papageorgakopoulos, G., Greenwell, H., Hill, M., Vidal, R. & Scheetz, J.P. (2008) Root coverage using an acellular dermal matrix and comparing a coronally positioned tunnel to a coronally positioned flap approach. *Journal of Periodontology*, **79**, 1022–1030.
31. Cummings, L.C., Kaldahl, W.B. & Allen, E.P. (2005) Histologic evaluation of autogenous connective tissue and acellular dermal matrix grafts in humans. *Journal of Periodontology*, **76**, 178–186.
32. Griffin, T.J., Cheung, W.S., Zavras, A.I. & Damoulis, P.D. (2006) Postoperative complications following gingival augmentation procedures. *Journal of Periodontology*, **77**, 2070–2079.
33. Livesey, S.A., Herndon, D.N., Hollyoak, M.A., Atkinson, Y.H. & Nag, A. (1995) Transplanted acellular allograft dermal matrix. Potential as a template for the reconstruction of viable dermis. *Transplantation*,**60**, 1–9.
34. Chambrone, L., Sukekava, F., Araujo, M.G., Pustiglioni, F.E., Chambrone, L.A. & Lima, L.A. (2010) Root-coverage procedures for the treatment of localized recession-type defects: A Cochrane systematic review. *Journal of Periodontology*, **81**, 452–478.
35. Henderson, R.D., Greenwell, H., Drisko C. *et al.*(2001) Predictable multiple site root coverage using an acellular dermal matrix allograft. *Journal of Periodontology*, **72**, 571–582.
36. Paolantonio, M., Dolci, M., Esposito, P. *et al.*(2002) Subpedicleacellular dermal matrix graft and autogenous connective tissue graft in the treatment of gingival recessions: A comparative 1-year clinical study. *Journal of Periodontology*, **73**, 1299–1307.
37. Tal, H., Moses, O., Zohar, R., Meir, H. & Nemcovsky, C. (2002) Root coverage of advanced gingival recession: A comparative study between acellular dermal matrix allograft and subepithelial connective tissue grafts. *Journal of Periodontology*, **73**, 1405–1411.
38. Woodyard, J.G., Greenwell, H., Hill, M. *et al.*(2004) The clinical effect of acellular dermal matrix on gingival thickness and root coverage compared to coronally positioned flap alone. *Journal of Periodontology*, **75**, 44–56.

39. Allen, E.P. (2010) Subpapillary continuous sling suturing method for soft tissue grafting with the tunneling technique. *The International Journal of Periodontics & Restorative Dentistry*, **30**, 479–485.

40. Sclar, A.G. (2003) The vascularized interpositional periosteal-connective tissue (VIP-CT) flap. In: A.G. Sclar (ed), *Soft Tissue and Esthetic Considerations in Implant Therapy*, pp. 163–188. Quintessence, Chicago, IL.

10 Future Potential for Minimally Invasive Periodontal Therapy

Stephen K. Harrel and Thomas G. Wilson Jr.

Based on the enthusiastic acceptance of nonsurgical treatment and minimally invasive surgery in medicine and dentistry, the future for the discipline in periodontal treatment is bright. As improvements in visualization technology come to the marketplace, a minimally invasive nonsurgical approach will likely become the routine first step in periodontal therapy. With diligence and expert application, many if not most periodontal therapy may likely be performed non-surgically. However, for the foreseeable future, there will almost certainly remain situations where surgical care will be necessary.

Goals and pitfalls of periodontal therapy

The basic tenants of periodontal therapy are unlikely to change no matter what physical approach is taken. There is almost universal agreement that periodontal diseases stem from the combination of microbiota and the body's response to these microbiota and their byproducts. Part of treatment will be to balance this dynamic system to limit the insult to the tissue. At present, personal oral hygiene is important to remove local etiologic factors, but we have very little influence on the systemic response. Without the body's defenses, we would rapidly lose teeth from periodontal diseases, and yet much of the destruction from periodontal diseases stems from this defense mechanism.

Minimally Invasive Periodontal Therapy: Clinical Techniques and Visualization Technology, First Edition.
Edited by Stephen K. Harrel and Thomas G. Wilson Jr.
© 2015 John Wiley & Sons, Inc. Published 2015 by John Wiley & Sons, Inc.
Companion Website: www.wiley.com/go/harrel/minimallyinvasive

Periodontal therapy whether through a traditional approach or a minimally invasive approach is a process of minimizing the risk factors for periodontal destruction, repairing the destruction that has already occurred, and once we have repaired the damage, to keep the process from reoccurring. At the heart of our therapy is the debridement of the root, the reduction of the microbiological load within the sulcus/pocket, and stimulating periodontal regeneration. This chapter will look at how these goals may be addressed in the future through a minimally invasive approach.

Nonsurgical therapy

There is a possibility that if the root surfaces could be completely debrided of calculus and biofilm, then "spontaneous" regeneration of periodontal tissues might result. When this is possible through a nonsurgical approach, surgical periodontal treatment could cease to be a necessity. The problem is that using traditional approaches in many instances, surgical access is currently necessary for complete debridement. The major problem facing nonsurgical periodontal therapy is the deficiencies in the current technology available for visualizing the pocket. A third generation of the glass fiber endoscope is scheduled for the introduction in the near future. This device will have the same basic technology as is currently available but will give a much clearer image. As mentioned in Chapter 2, the next step in improvement will most likely be the development of a miniature camera, similar to the one in the surgical videoscope but much smaller so that it can be placed into the intact sulcus/pocket. This is a technology that is available at this time but not currently economically practical. A videoscope for nonsurgical periodontal therapy will not change what is currently done with a glass fiber endoscope; but due to improved visualization, it should make the therapy much easier to perform.

Methods for the removal of root-borne deposits will also improve. One possible approach would be a device to detect calculus that could be used in combination with the videoscope. Wilson's study on the near-universal association of calculus with inflammation of the pocket wall clearly indicates that to be successful in our treatments, we must do a better job of calculus removal. One of our problems today is that we must rely on a less than perfect visual analysis of the root surface to determine where the calculus is located. We need a detection device that can differentiate between dentine, cementum, and calculus.

Once we know where the calculus is, we need to be able to remove it. The instruments we have now are extremely crude for the level of cleaning that needs to be performed. A small Gracey curette or traditional ultrasonic tip visualized with the videoscope appears huge compared to the islands of calculus on the root surface. The ideal would be an instrument that is associated with the calculus detector. This would allow the instrument to locate and remove the calculus while it was "in the sights." Prototypes of lasers have shown some success, but today's lasers are hopelessly crude and often destructive. It is possible that the laser energy could be generated in an electronic component at the tip of the instrument. Within this same context would be a microultrasonic that sent out a single burst of precision-guided energy. It is also possible that a form of energy that is not currently used in dentistry might be applied. The hammer effect of a piezoelectric crystal might also be possible. A dental piezoelectric scaler applies energy to a crystal in the scaler handle that is attached to the shaft of the scaler, and the energy is transferred to the tip of the scaler. It might be possible to apply a burst of current to a tiny peizo crystal at the end of a microprobe that gave a direct hammer action to the calculus that has been located by the detector probe. There is the potential for making this entire apparatus no larger than a periodontal probe. Many methods are possible, but active research will be necessary.

Surgical therapy

The anatomic configurations of root structure and bone loss will probably make surgical intervention necessary for regeneration in the foreseeable future. This is due to the inherent difficulty in accessing many of the sites where calculus forms on the root surfaces. With the videoscope, it is possible to visualize and access almost all areas of the root surfaces even when very small incisions are utilized. However, the currently available videoscope is too large to visualize most furcations that are more extensive than a class I; therefore, a smaller videoscope is needed. An ideal instrument size for surgical minimally invasive procedures would be approximately 0.5 mm in diameter. Again this is technically feasible at this time but is impractical to create. There is a strong likelihood that these difficulties can be overcome in the foreseeable future.

Minimally invasive surgery needs improved instruments for root and osseous defect debridement. Using the videoscope, anatomic irregularities and areas of calculus are visible that are normally impossible to see with other methods of visualization. Removing this calculus is possible but difficult with our current instrumentation. In addition, a new set of instruments for removal or smoothing of anatomical defects is needed. The videoscope reveals grooves and defects in cementum and dentine that have previously been unrecognized. The source of these defects is unknown. No matter their cause, they are almost always filled with calculus. Currently, the defects are removed with standard hand instruments, diamond-coated ultrasonic tips, or rotary instruments. All of these instruments are relatively crude and remove large amounts of apparently healthy root structure in the process of removing the root defect. What is needed is the development of instruments that can be applied in a much more selective manner than those currently available. Logically, these would be "micro" versions of the instruments currently used. Looking further, it may be possible to "heal" or fill in these defects with some variation of the methods currently being used in the recalcification of early carious lesions. Because recalcification technology for caries is itself in early development, the applicability of this or other techniques to the problems encountered in periodontal therapy is currently an unknown.

The removal of granulation tissue from periodontal defects through the small access afforded by minimally invasive surgery is another area that needs particular attention. Various mechanical instruments for the removal of granulation tissue have been developed in the past, but none have been fully satisfactory at removing tissue or were impractical for use with small incision techniques. These include sharpened ultrasonic curettes, rotary instruments, and lasers. There is some question as to how much granulation tissue needs to be removed for successful regeneration. One of the reasons given for removing granulation tissue is that it contains bacteria. While this is true, this can also be said for virtually all of the tissue surrounding a periodontal lesion both before and immediately after surgery. There is a good chance that to achieve healing, it is only necessary to remove enough granulation tissue to allow for debridement of the root surface. As visualization devices become smaller, we may find that removal of large amounts of granulation tissue becomes unnecessary.

Many regeneration techniques are well suited to the current minimally invasive surgical techniques. All of the liquid or semiliquid biologic agents such as enamel matrix proteins and recombinant bone morphogenic proteins are easily placed through small access opening. The same is true for most bone grafting materials that are in a granular form. The two current methods of regeneration that are not suitable for a minimally invasive approach are membranes for guided tissue regeneration and block grafting. The use of a block bone graft by its very nature does not lend itself to a minimally invasive approach. The use of a membrane is contraindicated where the incisions or flap reflection would have to be extended to allow for the placement of the membrane. The inability to use a membrane is not a major consideration because a membrane does not appear to be necessary for regeneration when the blood supply to the surgical area is spared with the use of minimally invasive surgery.

Goals for minimally invasive periodontal therapy

The long-term goals for minimally invasive periodontal therapy may well be a hybrid between nonsurgical and surgical minimally invasive treatment. It is conceivable that in the future, technology will allow for treatment of periodontal disease using incisions that are less damaging than is currently caused by placing a traditional curette into an intact periodontal pocket/sulcus. Such a minimally invasive technique might consist of inserting two medium-sized needles into the gingival tissue, possiblyone on the buccal and one on the lingual surface, and then performing all manipulations through these needles. One needle would allow for visualization; the other needle would allow for removal of calculus, smoothing of the roots, and placement of regenerative materials. While such a technique might be considered dreaming at this point, the technologic leap that is necessary to accomplish this or some other similar technique is less of a leap than the one that has brought us from a gingivectomy to a traditional approach for regenerative surgery. The technology that is now cutting edge for nonsurgical and surgical minimally invasive periodontal therapy will likely be viewed as crude in 30 years. The future for improvements in periodontal therapy is virtually limitless. The one thing that appears ensured is that procedures for treatment will become more effective and more minimally invasive.

Index

Note: Page numbers in *italics* refer to Figures; those in **bold** to Tables

Allen Microsurgical Elevator, 153, *154*
AlloDerm, soft tissue grafting, 151
alveolar ridge defect, 159–161, *160–161*
amelogenins
    delivery, 128
    minimally invasive surgical technique
        (MIST), 131, 133, 136
    modified MIST, 131, *132*, 136
    as regenerative material, 128, *130*
American Academy of Periodontology
        (AAP), periodontal disease
    case type II-III (early-to-moderate), 39
    case type III-IV (moderate-to-severe), 48
    case type IV (advanced/severe), 43
anesthetic-local *vs.* subgingival
        topical anesthetic, 60
Angles classification, class III bilateral, 39

bone grafting techniques, 78, 103, *160*, 168
bruxism, 39

CAF *see* coronally advanced flap (CAF)
calculus
    in chronic inflammatory
        periodontal disease, 20
    deposition, cementoenamel junction, 22
    detection, 166–7
    forms, 20
    micro islands, 93, *93*
    and probing depth, correlation, 22
    removal, 55–6
    on root surfaces *see* minimally invasive
        surgery (MIS)
    subgingival debridement procedures, 22
Castroviejo Needle Holder, 156–7
cement
    implant, 61, *108–9*
    peri-implantitis, 67
    peri-implant soft tissue, 67, *67*
    problem, 69–70
    removal, 70

Minimally Invasive Periodontal Therapy: Clinical Techniques and Visualization Technology, First Edition.
Edited by Stephen K. Harrel and Thomas G. Wilson Jr.
© 2015 John Wiley & Sons, Inc. Published 2015 by John Wiley & Sons, Inc.
Companion Website: www.wiley.com/go/harrel/minimallyinvasive

cervical enamel projections (CEPs)
    Grade I, *32, 32–3*
    Grade II, *32–3, 33*
    Grade III, *32, 33*
chronic unacceptable probing depths, 61
closed root planing, 3
coronally advanced flap (CAF), 145–6

demineratized cortical human bone
    allograft (DFDBA), 94–5, *95, 105, 115*
dental endoscopic technique
    cervical enamel projections (CEPs)
        Grade I, *32, 32–3*
        Grade II, *32–3, 33*
        Grade III, *32, 33*
    components
        Bilumen construction, 18
        camera/LED/controller, *15, 16*
        dental endoscope, 16–18, *17*
        dual Luer–Lock connectors, 18, *18*
        DV2 perioscopy system, 15, *16*
        endoscopic explorer tissue
            retraction shield, 19, *19*
        handpiece, 15, *16*
        perioscopy system, 15, *17*
        self-contained water delivery
            device, 19, *20*
        single-use disposable endoscopic
            sheath, 18, *18*
    dental endoscopy explorers, *31*
    diamond-coated ultrasonic
        instruments, 31, *31*
    ectopic enamel removal, 32
    enamel pearls, 34
    enamel projections, 32
    instruction
        explorer and ultrasonic
            instrument, 35, *36*
        medium-to-medium plus power, 35
        patient positioning, 35
        recommended training, 35
        in subgingival visualization, 35
        tray setup, *35*
    microvisual full-mouth
        debridement, 29, *30*
    two-handed technique, 27, *30*
    ultrasonic powered instruments, 30–31
    "view, instrument and view"
        technique, 27

dental endoscopy explorers, *31*
DFDBA *see* demineratized cortical
        human bone allograft (DFDBA)
diamond-coated ultrasonic instruments
    magnetostrictive diamond-coated
        ultrasonic inserts, 31, *31*
    scalers, *107*
Diamond Safety Tip, 91–3, *92*
dual Luer–Lock connectors, 18, *18*
DV2 perioscopy system
    color LCD video monitor, 15, *16*
    master control unit (MCU) camera, 15

ectopic enamel removal, 32, 34
EDTA *see* ethylenediaminetetracetic
    acid (EDTA)
enamel matrix derivative (EMD), 82,
    94–5, *95, 105, 115*
enameloplasty, 34, *34*
enamel pearl, 34, *106, 107*
End-Cutting Intrasulcular Knife, 153, *154*
endoscope *see also* nonsurgical
        endoscopic treatment
    advantages, 55–6
    anesthetic-local *vs.* subgingival
        topical anesthetic, 60
    calculus removal, 55
    diagnostic, 60
    implants, 61, *62*
    learning curve
        field of vision recognition, 56
        Gutta percha (GP), *59*
        healthy sulcus with enamel, *57*
        inflamed adjacent soft tissue, *57*
        mandibular molar furcation, *59*
        nondominant hand training, 56
        open margin (OM), *59*
        porcelain crown and root surface, *59*
        soft tissue and root surface, *57, 58*
        subgingival calculus, *58*
        subgingival deposits removal, 56
        vertical fracture, *58*
        void filling, *60*
    limitations, 61–2
    in pocket probing depth, 60–61
    in sulcus at CEJ level, *56*
    and videoscope
        blue-gray biofilm, 67, *67*
        bone loss, 68

cement, 67, *67*, 69–70
clinical and radiographic
  information gathering, 66
"granulation" tissue removal, 66
inflammatory lesion, 66
mandibular second molar
  abutment, 71–2, *72*
maxillary left central incisor, 73, *73–4*
osseointegrated implant, 70, *71*
peri-implant diseases, 66–9
periodic right-angle radiographs, 66
probing depths, 70–1
re-osseointegration, 67–8
single-unit cemented fixed
  partial denture, 70, *71*
subgingival calculus, 67
swelling complaint, 70
endoscopic explorer, 13
ethylenediaminetetracetic acid (EDTA)
  calculus removal, 93, *94*, *111*, *115*
  root preparation, *101*, *104*, *105*, 153

FGGs *see* free gingival grafts (FGGs)
free gingival grafts (FGGs), 143–5

gingivectomy, 145, 169

implant(s)
  abutment interface, 70
  endoscope, 61, *62*
  peri-implantitis infection, 37
internal mattress suture, modified MIST,
  128, 130, 133, *133*, *135*
intrabony defects
  classification, 123
  first lower molar, *137*
  minimally invasive surgical
    technique (MIST), 118, 131
  modified MIST, 118
  morphology and extension, 123
  pockets treatment, 122
  radiographic image, *124*, *128*,
    130, *133*, *134*

laser curettage, 38
laser pocket disinfection, 38
laser surgery, full-mouth
  azithromycin, 48
  implant placement, 48

laser tip view, 48, *50*
periodontal charting, 51
periodontal maintenance, 48
periodontal probing depths, 48, *50*
post restorative bridge upper
  anterior 9-11, 48, *50*
pre-Tx perio charting, 48, *49*
pre-Tx X-rays upper anterior bridge
  9-11, 48, *49*
radiograph, 48, *51*
ultrasonic endoscopic debridement, 48
upper anterior bridge, pre-Tx
  photo, 48, *48*
loupes *see* surgical telescopes (loupes)
luting agent, minimal, 70

magnetostrictive diamond-coated
  ultrasonic inserts, 31, *31*
microvisual full-mouth
  debridement, 29, *30*
Miller Class l recession sites, 151
"mini-flap", 78
minimally invasive periodontal therapy
  goals, 168–9
  microbiota combination, 165
  nonsurgical therapy, 166–7
  personal oral hygiene, 165
  risk factors minimization, 166
  surgical techniques
    bone grafting techniques, 78
    interproximal bone, 77
    "mini-flap", 78
    osseous surgery, 77
    periodontal tissue,
      regeneration, 77, 78
    pocket elimination/amelioration, 78
    root surfaces, debridement, 77
    vertical releasing incisions, 78
    Widman procedure, 77–8
  surgical therapy, 167–8
minimally invasive soft tissue grafting
  advantages, 157
  evolution
    coronally advanced flap (CAF), 145–6
    free gingival grafts (FGGs), 145
    gingivectomy, 145
    open vascular recipient bed, 145
    palatal donor tissue, 145
    root coverage, CTG procedure, 145–6

minimally invasive soft tissue
    grafting (*Cont'd*)
  indications
    attached gingiva, 143–4
    complete root coverage, 144
    dense collagenous connective
        tissue, 144
    exposed roots coverage, 144
    free gingival grafts (FGGs), 144
    gain of keratinized tissue, 144
    mucogingival junction (MGJ), 143–4
    subepithelial connective tissue
        graft (CTG) procedure, 144
  tunnel technique
    allograft donor tissue, 151–3
    allograft placement, 156
    intrasulcular site preparation, 153
    postoperative care, 157
    recipient site preparation, 146–50
    root preparation, 153
    suturing, 156–7
minimally invasive surgery (MIS), 82
  calculus on root surfaces
    EDTA, biomodification, *111*
    irregularities, *112*
    mechanical removal, *104*
    mid-lingual surface, *109*
    periodontal defect, deep
        calculus area, *110*
    smooth "burnished" calculus, *110*
    ultrasonic instruments
        and hand scalers, *111*
  case selection, 83–6
  cement, on implants, *108, 109*
  closed subgingival scaling, 82
  debridement
    biomodification,EDTA, 93, *94,
        101, 104, 105*
    calculus, micro islands, 93, *93*
    defect, 90–91
    Diamond Safety Tip, 91–3, *92*
    granulation tissue, removal, 90–91, *92*
    magnification, 91, *92*
    microcalculus removal, 93, *93*
    ultrasonic scaler, 91–2
    Younger-Goode 7/8 curette
        blade, 91, *91*
  enamel matrix derivative (EMD), 82
  granulation tissue removal, *100, 103, 104*

incision and flap design
    disposable microsurgical knifes, 88, *90*
    initial sulcular incisions, 87, *88*
    interproximal defect visualization,
        86, *86,* 87, *87*
    lingual access approaches, 86
    modified Orban knife, 87–8, *89, 90*
    osseous defect, 86
    push-pull cutting capabilities, 87, *89*
    routine pocket measurements, 86
    sulcular incisions, jointing, 87, *88*
  "lines" on root surfaces, *112–113*
  maxillary molar bifurcation defect,
        treatment, *114–115*
  nonsurgical treatment, 83
  palatal incision, periodontal defect, *102*
  periodontal defect, *99, 100*
  periodontal regeneration, 78
  pocket probing depth
    and CAL, 82
    chart, 83, *84*
  pocket probing depth, presurgical
        buccal view, 98, *98*
  postoperative instructions, 97
  post surgery, surgical area buccal
        view, *101, 102*
  presurgical lingual view, *99*
  presurgical pocket probing depths, 82
  quadrant charting, *84, 85*
  recession, 82
  regenerative materials
    demineratized cortical human bone
        allograft (DFDBA), 94–5, *95*
    enamel matrix derivative (EMD),
        94–5, *95*
    flaps, soft tissue healing, 94–5
    guided tissue regeneration, 95
    periodontal regeneration, 94–5
    Vicryl mesh, 95
  root abnormalities and diagnosis
    biomodification, *107*
    decay, *107*
    diamond-coated ultrasonic scalers, *107*
    enamel pearl, *106, 107*
    maxillary molar bifurcation
        defect, *105*
    pulp chamber, *108*
    root resorbtion, *106*
  small incision surgery, *85*

surgical principles
    blood supply preservation, 82–3
    minimum traumatic damage, 83
    split thickness dissection, 83
    suturing, 83
    un-incised tissue, cyanotic
        appearance, 83
suturing
    papilla tissues coronal, 96–7, *97*
    4-0 plain collagen, 96
    vertical mattress suture, 96, *96, 97*
videoscope, 82
visualization and magnification
    improvement, 86
minimally invasive surgical technique
    (MIST) *see also* periodontal
    regeneration
blood clot formation, 117–118
buccal and the lingual
    intrasulcular incisions
    amelogenins, regenerative
        materials, 131
    defect and residual bone
        crest, 126–8, *127–8*
    EDTA application, 131
    flap mobility, 128–131, *129–30*
    scaling and root planing, 131
buccal horizontal cut, 125
clinical indications and diagnostic
    procedures
    flap design, 124, *125*
    interproximal intrabony defect, 123
    intrabony defects, 123, *124*
    local anesthetic, 123
    nonsurgical cause-related
        therapy, 121–2
    papilla preservation flap, 125
    periodontal evaluation, 121, *122*
    periodontal probe, *123*
    topographic extension around
        teeth, 123
Cohort studies and randomized
    controlled clinical trials, 118–121,
    119, 120
defect-associated interdental papilla, 125
edema, 138
flap, primary closure, 138
interdental space width, 125
invasivity and patient side effects, 131

lingual/palatal incision, 126
mesio-distal extension, 126
microblade role, 126
modified MIST
    aggressive localized
        periodontitis, 131, *132–3*
    attention, 133
    buccal "surgical window," 133
    internal mattress suture, 133, *134–5*
    operative microscope/magnifying
        lenses, 133
modified papilla preservation
    technique (MPPT), 125, *126*
multiple intrabony defects
    treatment, 131
papilla preservation technique, 78–9
postoperative period and local
    side effects, 138
postsurgical protocols, 137
regeneration, 117–118
root hypersensitivity, 138
simplified papilla preservation flap
    (SPPF), 125, *126*
single modified internal mattress
    suture, 131
supportive periodontal care
    programs, 117
technical implications, 136
minimally invasive therapy, 1–2
MIST *see* minimally invasive surgical
    technique (MIST)
modified MIST *see* minimally invasive
    surgical technique (MIST)
modified papilla preservation
    technique (MPPT)
    minimally invasive surgical technique
        (MIST), 125, *126*
    regeneration, 118
mucogingival junction (MGJ), 143–4, 153

nonsurgical endoscopic treatment
    AAP case type IV (advanced/severe)
        periodontal disease, *43, 44*
    adjunctive antimicrobial agents, 38
    bone loss to apex, pre-Tx
        radiograph, *43, 44*
    doxycycline hyclate, 43
    gingivitis and periodontitis, 36
    inflammatory signs, clinical diagnosis, 37

nonsurgical endoscopic treatment (*Cont'd*)
  local anesthesia, 43
  mechanical debridement, 37–8
  minocycline HCl placement, 44, *44*
  objectives, 36
  peri-implantitis, 36–7
  peri-implant mucositis, 36
  periodontal disease treatment
    protocol, 38
  periodontal pathogens, 38
  pocketing, pre-treatment periodontal
    charting, *43*
  radiographic bone repair, post
    treatment X-ray, *45*
  systemic antibiotic therapy, 38
  topical anti-infective
    chemotherapeutics, 38
  ultrasonic endoscopic debridement
    periodontal charting, 39, *42*
    periodontal probing depths, 39
    post-Tx mandibular linguals, 39, *42*
    post-Tx photo, 39, *41*
    pretreatment panographic
      radiograph, *39*
    pre-Tx periodontal charting, 39, *40*
    pre-Tx photo facials, 39, *41*
  ultrasonic scaling, under local
    anesthetic, 45–8
nonsurgical sulcular debridement, 38

palatal donor
  allograft, 151
  site, 151, 157, *159*
  surgery, 151
  tissue, 144–6, *147*
palatal grafts *see* minimally invasive
    soft tissue grafting
peri-implant diseases, 36 *see also*
    endoscope
peri-implantitis, 36–7, 69
peri-implant mucositis, 36, 67, 68–9
periodontal disease treatment protocol, 38
periodontal osseous surgery, 77–8
periodontal regeneration
  blood clot formation, 117–118
  concepts, 118
  definition, 117
  demineratized cortical human bone
    allograft (DFDBA), 94–5, *95*
  enamel matrix derivative (EMD), 94–5, *95*

flap designs, 118
flaps, soft tissue healing, 94–5
guided tissue regeneration, 95
modified papilla preservation
    technique (MPPT), 118
periodontal regeneration, 94–5
regenerative material selection, 136, *137*
simplified papilla preservation
    flap (SPPF), 118
Vicryl mesh, 95
perioscopy system
  CCD/LED camera, 15
  medical grade monitor, 15, *17*
piezo scalers, 61
pocket elimination/amelioration, 78
pocket probing depth
  chart, *84, 85*
  dental implant and, 61
  endoscope, 60–61
  mean, 82
  periodontal disease examination, 23
  periodontal evaluation, 121
  presurgical, 82
  residual deep, 122
  subgingival calculus, 60–61
pocket sterilization, 38

root surfaces
  calculus on
    EDTA, biomodification, *111*
    irregularities, *112*
    mechanical removal, *104*
    mid-lingual surface, *109*
    periodontal defect, deep
      calculus area, *110*
    smooth burnished calculus, *110*
    ultrasonic instruments
      and hand scalers, *111*
  debridement, 77
  endoscopic evaluation, 22
  soft tissue and, *57, 58*
routine pocket measurements, 86

sheath, single-use disposable
    endoscopic, 18, *18*
simplified papilla preservation
    flap (SPPF)
  minimally invasive surgical
    technique (MIST), 125, *126*
  regeneration, 118

socket enhancement, *73, 73–4*
soft tissue grafting *see* minimally
       invasive soft tissue grafting
subepithelial connective tissue graft
       (CTG) procedure, 144
surgical microscope
   facial flap access, 9
   facial tissues handling, 9
   high magnification, 8
   inner ear surgery, 8
   installation, 8
   magnification and light, 9
   minimal disruption, 9
   MIST and M-MIST procedures, *8*
   periodontal plastic surgeries, 9
   in posterior and lingual areas, 9
   refocus, patient movement, 9
   soft tissue grafts placement, 8
   suturing of tissues, 9
surgical telescopes (loupes)
   advantages, 7
   disadvantages, 7–8
   focal length, 7
   halogen/LED light, 7
   integral light, 7
   magnification, 6
   range, 6–7
surgical videoscope *see also* endoscope
   blood and surgical debris, 10
   carbon fiber retractor, 10
   external camera, 9
   gas shielding device, 11, *11*
   image transfer to monitor, 9
   kidney, nonsurgical exploration, 10
   modifications, 10
   periodontal defect, buccal/lingual
       aspect, 10
   root abnormalities and diagnosis
       biomodification, *107*
       decay, *107*
       diamond-coated ultrasonic scalers, *107*
       enamel pearl, *106, 107*
       maxillary molar bifurcation
           defect, *105*
       pulp chamber, *108*
       root resorbtion, *106*
   small incision surgeries, 11
   stainless steel tube, 9
   videoscope-assisted minimally invasive
       surgery (V-MIS), 10, *10, 11*

traditional scalers and ultrasonics, 61
tunnel technique, soft tissue grafting
   allograft donor tissue
       acellular dermal matrix
           (ADM), 151
       advantage, 151
       AlloDerm, 151
       keratinized tissue gain, 151–3, *152*
       limitation factors, 151
       Miller Class l recession sites, 151
       palatal donor site, 151
   allograft placement, *155, 156*
   allografts, 146
   free gingival graft (FGG), 143
   intrasulcular site preparation,
       153, *154*
   palatal donor tissue, 146, *147*
   postoperative care, 157
   recipient site preparation
       "biologic width", 146
       disadvantages, 150
       interdental embrasure space, 148
       intrasulcular incisions, 146
       maxillary arch, root
           exposure, 148, *148*
       papillary incisions, indications,
           149, *149–50*
       vertical incisions elimination, 150
   ridge augmentation
       alveolar ridge defect, 159–161,
           160–161
       papillary areas and edentulous
           ridge areas, 159
       pediculated palatal connective
           tissue graft harvest, 158, *159*
       rotated palatal pedicle graft
           technique, 158
       VIP-CT grafting technique, 158
   root coverage grafting, 146
   root preparation, 153, *154–5*
   suturing, 156–7

ultrasonic endoscopic periodontal
       debridement
   antibiotics, 23
   computerized charting
       program, 23, 27
   dental endoscopy, 14
   fiber-optic illumination, 14
   full-mouth laser surgery, 48–52

ultrasonic endoscopic periodontal
  debridement (*Cont'd*)
  indications
    components, 15–19
    DV2 perioscopy system, 15
    patients, 15
  magnifications, 14
  microvisual approach, 13
  minimally invasive procedures, 13
  nonsurgical endoscopic treatment
    selection, 36–9
  periodontal endoscope, 13
  perioscopy system, *14*
  pocket probing depths, 23–6
  real-time video, 13
  subgingival environment
    advantage, 20
    blind scaling and root planing, 23
    bright fiber-optic illumination, 20
    calculus deposits removal, 20
    cementoenamel junction, calculus
      deposition, 22
    chronic inflammatory periodontal
      disease, 20, 23
    closed scaling and root planing, 22
    endoscope probe, 19
    factors affecting instrumentation, 21
    gingival wall, 19–20
    goal, 22
    hand instrumentation and
      ultrasonics combination, 22
    oral cavity, ecological niches, 22
    periodontal pathogens, 22
    residual calculus and probing depth,
      correlation, 22
    root surfaces, endoscopic
      evaluation, 22
    scaling and root planing, 19, *21*, 22
technique, endoscopic *see* dental
  endoscopic technique
treatment and follow-up
  fifteen months post
    micro-ultrasonic, 27, *28*
  post treatment X-ray, 27, *29*
  post-Tx X-ray, 27, *30*
  pretreatment X-ray, 27, *28*, *29*

ultrasonic scaling, under local
    anesthetic
  amoxicillin and metronidazole, 45
  periodontal charting, 45, *47*
  pocket depths reduction, 48
  povidone-iodine application, 45
  pretreatment periodontal
    charting, 45, *46*
  radiograph, 45, *46*, *47*

Vascularized Interpositional
    Periosteal-Connective Tissue
    Graft (VIP-CT), 158
Vicryl mesh, 95
videoscope-assisted minimally invasive
    surgery (V-MIS), 10, *10*, *11*, 81–2
    see also minimally invasive
    surgery (MIS)
visualization, minimally invasive
    periodontal therapy
  closed root planing procedures
    blood and debris removal, 6
    camera, 6
    clarity of image, 5–6
    glass fiber endoscope, *4*, 4–5
    nonsurgical, 6
    periodontal endoscope, 4–5
    routine periodontal treatments, 5
    single-use sterile disposable
      sheath, 5, *5*
    smaller fibers uses, 6
  periodontal surgery, 4
  root planing, 3
  subgingival scaling, 3
  surgical microscope, 8–9
  surgical telescopes (loupes), 6–8
  surgical videoscope, 9–11

Widman procedure, 77–8

Younger-Good 7/8 curette
  allograft placement, *155*, 156
  graft insertion, *155*, 156
  granulation tissue removal, 91, *91*, 100
  interdental alveolar crest
    elevation, 153, *154*